Brown County Public Library
205 Locust Lane / P.O. Box 8
Nashville, IN 47448
Telephone & TDD (812) 988-2850
FAX (812) 988-8119

New York Times Bestselling Author

JANE VELEZ-MITCHELL
AND SANDRA MOHR

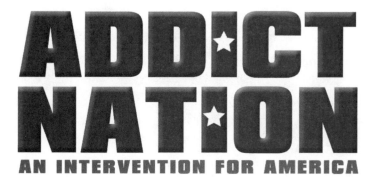

ADD★CT NAT★ON

AN INTERVENTION FOR AMERICA

Health Communications, Inc.
Deerfield Beach, Florida

www.hcibooks.com

Library of Congress Cataloging-in-Publication Data

Velez-Mitchell, Jane.
    Addict nation : an intervention for America / Jane Velez-Mitchell and
Sandra Mohr.
        p. cm.
    Includes bibliographical references and index.
    ISBN-13: 978-0-7573-1545-9
    ISBN-10: 0-7573-1545-3
    1. Compulsive behavior.   I. Mohr, Sandra.   II. Title.
    RC533.V45 2010
    362.196'85227—dc22

                                                                    2010046514

Publisher: Health Communications, Inc.
              3201 S.W. 15th Street
              Deerfield Beach, FL 33442-8190

Cover design: Liz Bolwell
Hair and makeup stylist: Jill DeVito
Cover photographer: Andrew Brucker
Photo stylist: Jannette Patterson
Interior design and formatting by Dawn Von Strolley Grove

For

Ingrid Newkirk
whose limitless compassion and tireless campaigning
for the world's most oppressed creatures
is a beacon of hope that
evolution toward kindness is possible.

CONTENTS

ACKNOWLEDGMENTS

Working with Carol Rosenberg, HCI's editor extraordinaire, has been a true gift. With enormous skill and understanding, she has guided Sandra and me through the process of making a complex premise relatable. We are also forever grateful to HCI president and publisher Peter Vegso for his confidence in our ideas and his willingness to give us a dynamic platform to express them. The entire HCI team, especially Kim Weiss, deserve kudos for getting the word out about this project. Our literary agent, Sharlene Martin, is a fierce champion of our ideas who encouraged us to tell this story. My news agent Carole Cooper has always been there for me as a friend and wise mentor.

Thanks also to the amazing team at HLN for the very rare and precious opportunity to express opinions that are fresh and controversial before a worldwide audience. I will always be in gratitude to Ken Jautz, executive vice president of CNN, who gave me my big break by hiring me for the HLN show *Issues*. I am also thrilled to be working for Scot Safon, executive vice president for CNN Worldwide in charge of HLN, who has encouraged me to give voice to my passions. My thanks as well to Bill Galvin, HLN senior vice president, who has being a real champion. My executive producer Stephanie Todd is not only a dynamic leader but a friend who has given me the confidence to take risks. I am in debt to the entire *Issues* team, especially Jennifer Williams, Rob Beck, Emily Barsh, Kaylin Rocco, Sarah Carden, Katy Rogers, Annette Smith, Amy

Doyle, Cameron Baird, Alicia Johnson, Amanda Sloane, and Jackie Taurianen. They all use their considerable expertise to bring my rough ideas into sharp focus. Carolyn Disbrow of CNN public relations has also been incredibly supportive. Nancy Grace and her EP Dean Sicoli have also always been there for me. Finally, Liz Bolwell has been a true rock for Sandra and me as we navigated our way through the minefields of America's addictive habits. Her patience, wisdom, and humor are extraordinary.

"The most exquisite paradox . . .
as soon as you give it all up,
you can have it all."

–Ram Dass

INTRODUCTION:
Why This Book Will Change Your Life

The other night I went to a charity event at a sprawling private home in the hills of Los Angeles. I parked in front of a house down the block, got out of the car, and found myself staring at a distinctive front door. With a start, I realized, "Hey, that's the place I hit bottom fifteen years ago." Yep, it was through that fancy door that I was carried out of that house over someone's shoulder . . . in an alcoholic blackout. I remembered the house only because a friend of mine had lived there and I had visited it often . . . until that wild, out-of-control night.

It was great to be confronted by that memory because it put in sharp relief how much better my life has become in the decade and a half that I've been sober. Standing there in the near darkness, those crazy years when my drinking was out of control sped through my mind like a movie stuck in fast forward.

As I walked away and headed toward the party where a chic Hollywood crowd was gathering, I felt immense gratitude. I no longer had to worry about what inappropriate thing I might do or say as the night wore on. I knew that the next day I would remember everything that happened at the party. I knew I would not have to phone anyone the next morning for a "damage assessment," nor would I have to apologize for anything I did or said. There would be no embarrassment or remorse or worry. In other words, I felt

1

completely free. More than anything else, that's what sobriety is: FREEDOM!

Why am I telling you this? Because I want *you* to experience that same freedom! Right now you might be thinking, *The nerve of that Jane, to assume whoever's reading this book is an alcoholic!* No, I'm not jumping to that conclusion, but I am making a pretty safe bet that you *are* an addict. Why? Because virtually everyone in America is hooked on something. We are a nation of addicts! In *Addict Nation*, you'll learn how you and I, and other Americans, are being lured into a slew of addictions that are supremely self-destructive. They're making us high. They're making us overweight. They're keeping us constantly distracted. They're trivializing our most important relationships. They're putting us in debt. And they're destroying our natural world. We're all becoming slaves to our worst impulses. We are giving up our freedoms.

Sadly, what's happening is the exact opposite of what our Founding Fathers had in mind. The United States of America was created precisely to celebrate "life, liberty, and the pursuit of happiness." Freedom of choice is the underlying premise of our society. That means we get to decide how we live our lives, how we spend our money, what we eat and wear, and how we relax in our "free" time.

I love the freedoms I have as an American, and I never take them for granted. In fact, that's why I've written this book. It's crucial that we Americans confront the huge addiction epidemic that is robbing us of our ability to make rational choices in our own true self-interest.

Enslavement comes in many different forms. It's not always someone pointing a gun at you or building a wall to keep you where you are. There is also psychological and emotional bondage. If you know intellectually that you are on the verge of making a bad choice, and, still, you cannot stop yourself, then you are just as enslaved as if somebody were pointing a gun at you. Either way, you do not have what it takes to say no to self-defeating behavior.

Addiction Is Determining Our Behavior

We're all familiar with the obvious addictions: drugs and alcohol. Those obsessions have been with us since Adam first met Eve. They plucked their first grapes and discovered the mind-altering beverage that resulted from the fermentation process. There's even the occasional reference to alcoholism in the Bible. Addictions have gone forth and multiplied since biblical times. We now have many more temptations to seduce us into dangerous and even deadly choices. Symbolically, the snake may have first starred in the role of pusher by beguiling Eve into eating the apple, who passed it to Adam, getting them both thrown out of Eden. Today, there are many complex forces, not unlike that serpent, which beguile us into bad behavior for their own purposes—usually for profit and power.

Increasingly, almost everything being presented to us as a "free choice" is being packaged and sold in a way that's designed to get us hooked in order to guarantee that we keep coming back for more. To offer just one obvious example, there's increasing evidence that fast food is addictive, which would go a long way toward explaining our obesity crisis. The psychologically addictive component is the constant drumbeat of advertizing to encourage fast food consumption, combined with its easy availability. The physically addictive component is fast food's high levels of sugar, salt, and fat, ingredients now being tied to compulsive consumption.[1]

For another example, one need look no further than our current foreclosure mess. Mortgages were offered to millions of people who really couldn't afford them. Predatory mortgage brokers got their cut and didn't seem to care what happened to the house or the home-owner after they sealed the deal. These seductive lending policies triggered an addictive binge of spending and overconsumption as people who bought homes above their means proceeded to furnish them using high-interest-rate credit cards. Eventually the house of (easy credit) cards crumbled. We were culturally intoxicated on a cocktail of complex lies, and now we're all reeling from the hang-over. All except the very rich, that is. They just keep getting richer, as America's wealth divide continues to widen. In almost every case, there is huge money to be made on seducing you into addictive behavior. Ask yourself, *Do I really want to be a slave, existing just to make someone else rich and powerful?* No, you say? Well, then, read on.

Freedom of choice implies that you have the free will to make a rational choice. Freedom of choice implies you are capable of deciding what is in your true self-interest. Addiction messes with that equation. Addiction, by definition, is being powerless to say no to a particular substance or behavior that generally gives you a quick hit of pleasure, but which often results in long-term pain or other negative consequences.

The Big Issue Is Addiction

Virtually every story I cover on my HLN TV show *Issues with Jane Velez-Mitchell* is, in some way, shape, or form about addiction. Let's examine some of the biggest stories of our time. In each case, the BIG ISSUE is addiction.

Michael Jackson, Anna Nicole Smith, DJ AM, Heath Ledger . . . these are just a few of the tragic headliners who've showcased the nation's epidemic of prescription drug addiction. There's even a hit show for high-profile drug addicts: *Celebrity Rehab with Dr. Drew.* Kirstie Alley has become the national symbol for our collective battle with obesity. She spilled her guts about her rollercoaster ride down and up the scale to Oprah, who could relate because she too has waged a long and very public losing battle with her weight. Could these two supertalented women perhaps be addicted to food? With nineteen kids and counting, the Duggars are clearly hooked on making babies . . . and getting on television. Ditto for the Octomom, plus John and Kate. With a baker's dozen of alleged mistresses, is it really a stretch to wonder if Tiger Woods was hooked on sex?

Okay, those are all famous people. So what? Do you really think stars are the only ones who grapple with compulsions like serial infidelity, overpopulation, pill popping, and gluttony? No. The only difference between stars and the rest of us is . . . their addictive behavior seems somehow more glamorous, more fascinating. And we all get to watch.

Addiction Often Comes Packaged as a Harmless Distraction

What's surpassed baseball as our number-one national pastime? Crime. America's extreme fixation on violence and murder has reached epidemic proportions. A beautiful Tennessee TV news anchorwoman is raped and murdered while minding her own business in her own home, a Georgia mom is abducted while walking down a country road near her parents' house, a little girl is kidnapped near a bus stop in California and held for eighteen years while her captor rapes her repeatedly, fathering two children by her. It seems every day brings a new horror story. And we're hooked! We want to know every last detail!

On my show *Issues,* I talk about our culture of violence and insist that, as we cover these stories, we analyze the root societal causes of crime and look for solutions lest we become just another showcase for the pornography of violence. Ironically, addiction itself is one of the most common causes of crime. People who are drunk or high on drugs are capable of monstrous violence they would never even consider while sober and often rob to support their habit. In fact, the title of this book came out of a recurring segment on my show called "Addict Nation," where my expert panel and I discuss how addiction is the underlying theme of so much disturbing news.

America's crime addiction can be seen in our obsession with the mass shooting du jour and the wild televised car chases. We all know how those car chases end. The suspect is always caught. Yet, we remain glued to the live coverage, drinking in the "suspense." After drugs, booze, and food, crime is perhaps our most potent and pervasive form of escape. You may now be thinking, *What's wrong with a little escapism? Is that really an addiction?*

Escapism is the root cause of all addiction. The motive for any addictive behavior is always the same: to stuff down and escape painful feelings and unpleasant truths by altering one's mental and emotional state with the addictive substance/behavior. Addiction is all about altering reality by "using" to tweak one's mood. The drug of choice may vary from addict to addict, but the purpose of using is always the same. Different addicts drive different cars, but they're all heading to the same destination. Oblivion.

Human beings are capable of becoming addicted to virtually anything—from plastic surgery to tattoos to texting. I can tell you from personal experience that addictions jump from one substance to another. When I gave up booze—voila, sugar popped up to take its place as my new obsession. Over the years, I've given up alcohol, drugs, sugar, meat, dairy, diet soda, violent movies, and a variety of other bad habits. But new addictions just keep cropping up. That's because all the behavior is driven by the same motive: to "check out," to numb, and to escape.

You're an addict when your behavior turns into a never-ending cycle of craving, bingeing, remorse, and withdrawal. That hangover, or withdrawal, then triggers a new bout of craving, and the cycle begins again.

Here's one of my addictive cycles. Every night when I leave work, I feel the urge to eat something. No problem there. It's what I crave that's the problem. As a vegan, I'm pretty much locked in to a healthy diet. You have to search long and hard to find vegan junk food. But, hey, I'm an addict. I will do that! I will systematically hunt down the most fattening, vegan dessert available anywhere in the tristate area. When I find it, I eat it quickly, voraciously, looking over my shoulder as if somebody will take it away from me if I don't gobble it down fast. About five minutes after the last bite, the remorse kicks in. *Why did I just do that? Didn't I just devour the same amount of calories it takes me an hour and a half to burn off during a session of thinly disguised torture called "hot" yoga? Why couldn't I have just had another serving of cantaloupe instead?*

Sometimes addiction is called "taking our comfort." When I'm eating the cake, a voice in my head tells me, "I'm entitled, I've earned it. I've worked hard all day. And it tastes so good! Damn the consequences!" When I get into the remorse phase minutes later, another voice in my head says, "Who was that person who wolfed down that vegan cake faster than you can say *organic fair-trade agave nectar*?" As an addict, I have a committee living in my head whose members love to argue and wage power plays.

Ultimately, I have had to counteract that addiction by simply giving up sweets entirely, even so-called healthy sweets like maple syrup, molasses, and, yes, agave nectar. Now I identify myself as "an alcoholic and a sugar addict." Being an addict, it's easier for me to give up the addictive substance entirely rather than try to negotiate with it. Bye-bye added sugar in all its forms. I simply cannot do sugar or booze in moderation. Put another way, I cannot use those substances successfully.

Any addiction is ultimately self-destructive, even an addiction to something that—in moderation—is good for you, like exercise.

So what kind of behavior is considered okay? What's not? It depends on the cultural norms of the moment. Suddenly, we've got pot stores popping up all over California and Colorado. The baby boomers, most of whom smoked pot as teens, grew up, got into power, and decided, "Come on, there are more important battles to wage than trying to stop people from lighting up, especially if they're sick and need some pain relief." Society is constantly reassessing its tolerance for certain addictive behaviors, declaring war on some addictions while encouraging others.

Remember the sixties? "If you can . . . you weren't there," is the tired joke. The sixties positively romanticized the use of psychedelics. Then the nineties demonized them. The fifties was one long love affair with smoking. By the nineties, cigarettes were considered gross, inspiring attitudes like "I could never date someone who smokes!" The disco seventies, where hot pants and platform shoes were the rage, looked askance on obesity. Today, there's an ill-advised fat acceptance movement. Our culture has lost its tolerance for drunks and smokers, but we still rationalize obesity as a lifestyle choice. Being morbidly overweight is an addiction to food, just like smoking is an addiction to cigarettes and getting drunk is an addiction to alcohol. To accept obesity unquestioningly is really to be an enabler of the problem.

Whether it's the neighbors' annual Oscar party, or Karaoke Wednesdays, human beings are pack animals. We move in groups from one behavioral landscape to another. We're always adjusting to the shifting sands of cultural attitudes. Simply put, America lurches from addiction to addiction, stamping out one bad habit only to see others take its place.

When Enough People Are Hooked, It Crosses the Line into a Social Contagion

Our entire nation is addicted to a slew of self-destructive, compulsive actions. You may be thinking, *Well, that's why we have the government, the media, and—yes—even big business. They help us fight these terrible social plagues.* FUHGEDDABOUDIT! The media, the government, and business are often the enablers ... even the pushers! The media relays and popularizes the bad habit, the government subsidizes it, and big business squeezes a buck out of it.

When somebody's absolutely got to have something, that's called demand. Addiction creates enormous demand, and there are massive profits in supplying what we crave.

The More Widespread an Addiction Gets, the More It Seems Normal

An extreme example of a dysfunction that has become accepted as normal in one part of the world is the burka women are forced to wear in some parts of the Middle East. I once had to try on a burka as part of a news story I was doing on the oppression of women. The second I put it on I felt like I was drowning. I couldn't see to the left or right of me. God help me if I had tried to cross the street. I probably would have been sideswiped by a bus. It was torture. I kept it on for three or four minutes, and then I just couldn't take it anymore. I ripped that freakin' burka off, threw it on the floor, and thanked heaven that I was born in America and not in the hills of Afghanistan. The burka is beyond oppressive. It's lunacy! But for the Taliban, it is their "normal."

Similarly, in America, self-destructive compulsions, like violent crime, war, overconsumption, overpopulation, prescription drug abuse, food addiction, Internet porn, and obsessive use of antibacterials are so widespread as to seem "normal." So we accept the behavior and cease to put it through our normal screening process. The bad habit gets a pass because "everybody's doing it!"

On *Issues,* I bring attention to the horrors of cultural addictions like overconsumption. However, I am often left disillusioned. Some of the smartest people I encounter don't seem at all bothered by America's pathological wastefulness. They react like there's something a little strange about me that I'm so concerned. Why? As we know, addiction can afflict anyone regardless of their income, education, or intelligence. America's best and brightest, despite their brains and positions of privilege, are also addicts, hooked on the very same social addictions as the rest of us! And, because they're smart, they can whip up the best excuses to justify our worst lifestyle choices.

If I go out to a fancy restaurant with a successful New York executive, the chances are that a good percentage of the food that comes to our table will be discarded. It's fashionable to order food and not eat much of it. Successful people do this all the time. Many women, especially, are brought up to never finish the last bite. If they leave half the plate, they feel even more refined. It's part of the mentality that you can never be too rich or too thin. As I watch the waiter take away a plate of barely eaten food, along with the rolls of untouched bread in the basket, all destined for the garbage bin, I think of a recent study. It says America could feed over 200 million adults every year, just with the food that ends up in our garbage cans. As we speak, 1 billion people are going hungry worldwide, according to the United Nations.[2] While my more successful friends certainly feign concern over that jaw-dropping imbalance, they actually seem more disturbed by my newest quirk. Now, when I go out to a restaurant, I take all the uneaten bread from the basket in the center of the table with me when I leave. I either give it to a homeless person or feed it to the hungry birds I'm always passing on the street. Apparently, this makes me a freak.

Maybe they're not so smart after all. This wastefulness is part and parcel of the addiction of overconsumption. We're hoarding for ourselves more than we can ever possibly consume, while others starve. It's obscene. But nobody is addressing the addictive nature of this behavior.

The Most Dangerous Addictions Are the Ones We Fail to Even Diagnose as Addictive Behavior

If you have an undiagnosed addiction, it's like not knowing you have a fatal cancer growing inside you. You're flying blind. You can't combat a problem until you correctly diagnose it. Right now, America is misdiagnosing some of its biggest problems, like obesity, materialism, and crime. It's no wonder they're just getting worse!

One thing we know about addicts: they don't listen to reason. A craving is a very powerful thing that has a force of its own like a hurricane or a tsunami. Have you ever tried to get a friend to stop smoking by telling them they're liable to get cancer? Ha! Reason is no match for a full-blown addiction. This is why addicts are known for being stubborn and defiant when somebody tries to stop them. When you scold a drunk for drinking too much, they're apt to storm out of the house and head toward the nearest bar. Well, the same thing applies to our social addictions like crime, materialism, excessive cleanliness, and gluttony. This is precisely why Americans keep getting fatter as we lecture everyone about the dangers of junk and fast food.

When It Comes to Combating Addictive Behavior, We Are Wasting Taxpayer Dollars Trying to Engineer Strictly Political Solutions

Politics is tone deaf to the psychological and emotional under-pinnings of America's worst problems, even as it throws billions of dollars at them. If you give a heroin junkie a wad of cash, it's not going to help him kick his habit. *Au contraire.*

Our healthcare debate is a perfect example. We keep talking about getting everybody insured. How about tackling the root cause of so much of the illness in America? Addiction! Overconsumption of alcohol is tied to an increased risk of breast cancer. The addiction there is alcoholism. Smoking has long been the nation's number-one preventable killer. Smoking is an addiction. And now obesity is creeping up and could ultimately surpass smoking as the country's leading preventable killer. Obesity is the result of food addiction.

Nobody's talking about this. If the government took better aim at those preventable killers, we might all be willing to embrace universal health insurance because it wouldn't be so damn expensive!

The same concept applies to America's other big issues, like prescription drug abuse, sexual exploitation, pollution, poverty, over-population, even crime and war. We must recognize that addiction is at the heart of these problems. We—as a culture—are hooked on these malignancies.

Addicts Have the Ultimate Sense of Entitlement— Nothing Will Stop Them From Getting Their Drug of Choice! That's the Addict Mind-Set

We can define *addiction.* It has certain clear-cut characteristics:

- an endless cycle of craving, bingeing, remorse, and withdrawal;

- a progressive pattern, leading to invariably uglier and more destructive behavior until a "bottom" is hit;
- obsessive rituals and elaborate paraphernalia;
- defiance and denial in the face of evidence of the wreckage caused by the addiction;
- strenuous and imaginative rationalizations to justify the addictive behavior;
- the "user" is invariably paired with a "pusher." One is exploited while the other profits.

Addiction spawns its own unique culture. In every addict's world, there is the "pusher" and, beyond, the "cartel," which reaps the profit. This even applies to chardonnay. Back when I was drinking, I felt like I was personally supporting the entire economy of France! My American Express bill was so heavy I did bicep curls with it. Opening the bill, I would have terrifying flashbacks of yelling, "Champagne for everyone!"

Addictions Are Expensive

That holds true for our national addictions to crime, war, sexual exploitation, animal exploitation, cleanliness, overconsumption, materialism, drugs, and food. In each of these categories, there are billions, if not trillions, of dollars at stake. Anyone who seeks to expose the addictions at the heart of these problems will provoke the wrath of powerful industries and government bureaucracies that perpetuate the status quo for their own gain.

If there were no prisons, what would happen to those corporations, unions, and government bureaucrats whose sole purpose is to supply and police those prisons? One of America's biggest "growth industries" is private prisons and related companies that have discovered a way to "cash in" on arresting, prosecuting, housing, feeding, and clothing inmates. How can they keep "growing" their business? By creating more criminals of course. (I will explain in one of the following chapters precisely how they do this.)

Hollywood also profits off of our culture of violence, selling the American public tickets to highly stylized assaults, car chases, rapes, and murders, glamorizing it all in the process.

Food addiction is making billions for fast-food manufacturers and agri-businesses that are protected by their allies in the U.S. Department of Agriculture (USDA) and subsidized by the U.S. government.

War addiction is fueled by the military-industrial complex. The Halliburtons and the Blackwaters make the news, but many mainstream companies also profit magnificently from war.[3]

Prescription drug addiction is encouraged by the secretive but powerful pharmaceutical industry that controls government decisions through its powerful lobby.

In all of the above cases, the people funding these powerful interests are you and me . . . the taxpayers and consumers. We, the people, are doubly exploited and victimized. We have to live with the albatross of addiction, and we make our enslavers rich in the process! It's a really bad deal.

Ironically, if all us consumers/taxpayers joined forces to demand change, we, as a unit, would be more powerful than the most powerful industrial cartels. But first the American people have to "hit bottom" on these cultural addictions and feel the desire to change!

Addiction Is Progressive

A fundamental truth of addiction is that if it's not confronted and treated, it will invariably get worse. That's because the addict's pleasure receptors become skewed and require an ever-increasing amount of the same substance/behavior for the high to kick in. In other words, addicts are insatiable and will always need more of their "junk" to get off and to stay high. So the addict's predicament is always getting more perilous.

In this book, I will offer you a view into our world from an addict's perspective and suggest where we might be headed. If you think things are bad now, imagine an America even more defined by life-threatening obesity, pervasive drug dependency, insatiable sexual perversion, ever more sadistic crime, widespread incarceration, and unnecessary war. That's where we are headed. I cover all these stories on my show *Issues,* and I see firsthand how it's all getting worse!

Do we really want a nation filled with citizens who are overwhelmingly obese, drug addicted, hooked on porn, and either criminally minded or potential victims? Do we really want to live in an America where a huge swath of our national resources is spent on incarcerating our own citizens and waging war on nameless, faceless strangers in foreign lands?

The choice is ours. *Addict Nation* is designed to be a blueprint for change. But first, we need to wake up to what's happening.

This is an intervention!

Chapter One
THE STUFFERS: Addicted to Consumption

-- -- -- -- -- -- -- -- -- -- --

N ot so long ago, simplicity was thrust upon me in a most bizarre and delightful way. I was sitting at my dining room table sipping a cup of French roast coffee with steamed soymilk. It was a typical foggy morning in the little beach community just south of Venice, California, which I called home. I was so close to the ocean that I could hear the waves break from where I sat. That sound has always been a comfort, reminding me of nature's omnipresence.

That autumn morning I happened to be at a crossroads. I was between jobs and relationships and wondering what to do next. Sitting there, staring at nothing in particular, I was surprised to see a text come in on my cell phone saying that I should expect a call from a network executive at any moment. I perked up and began staring at my cell phone.

In short order, the phone rang. A delightful voice on the other end of the line offered me a job hosting my own national TV show. Oh, and by the way, I'd have to start right away, as in that very minute. I would do the show in Los Angeles that same night and then fly to New York to begin working there two days later. Wow! Now that's quite a wake-up call! And it would prove to be in many ways.

I was thrilled and immediately said yes! It was like a gift from heaven. My eighteen years of living in Los Angeles came to an abrupt end, and life took me on its next adventure.

I packed two suitcases full of business jackets, pants, and blouses, t-shirts, pullovers, jeans, sneakers, and undies, plus a fall and winter coat. I tossed in my laptop, my iPod, a small iPod speaker, my file of bills and receipts, a few personal papers, plus some makeup and hairbrushes. My two rescue dogs went to the vet and got their travel papers, and the three of us hopped on a jet to Nueva York. Once there, we took a cab to my mom's apartment in midtown, the very apartment where I grew up.

I suddenly found myself back in my old bedroom where I had morphed from half pint to terrible teen. It contained a twin bed, a writing table, and a nightstand with a small TV set. It would turn out that, at ninety-four, my mother finally needed somebody to live with her. Also, my dogs—extraordinarily spoiled and prone to harmonically synchronized howling when left alone—were thrilled to have a doting grandma to play with while I was at work. As an added bonus, my mom happens to live conveniently close to the HLN studios where my show is broadcast. So I decided I really didn't need my own apartment just yet.

It didn't take me long to start noticing something else quite shocking. All that stuff I had left in LA? I really didn't miss it. I got rid of my car. I certainly didn't need to ship a vehicle to New York City. It was actually a relief not to have the responsibility of a car for the first time in decades. No car insurance for one. No trips to the dealership for tune-ups. No fender benders. No hunting for a parking spot. No stops at the gas station. No garages. No speeding tickets. Yippee! Not having a car frees up a lot of time and money. I also didn't miss that fancy big-screen TV I had left behind. It used to seduce me into watching way too many movies.

It would turn out that I had almost everything I needed to feel comfortable: my favorite music, my hookup to the Internet, and my mom's countless books. A health food store a few blocks away would keep me supplied with the sage and lavender oils that I love to luxuriate in. I also picked up a few vanilla-scented soy candles and some sticks of pine incense. It didn't take much for my room to feel, smell, and sound just like home. Right there, that taught me something. What makes a home isn't the stuff. It's the sensations, the feelings, and the companionship of the people and animals we love that allow us to identify a certain place as "home."

This whole experience led me to question my old assumptions about what I "needed" to own. Circumstances had forced me to leave most of my possessions behind, and something magical happened. With less stuff, I began feeling more "right sized." I felt freer, more mobile, more independent, less distracted by the responsibility of taking care of possessions. The feeling was intoxicating. It reminded me of the "pink cloud" I felt when I first got sober from alcohol years earlier. I had long suspected there was an addictive component to all the stuff I had accumulated over the course of my life: golf clubs that I never used, exercise equipment (that served as a very expensive clothes rack), and dozens of knick-knacks that started out as decorations and ended up as clutter. This experience of suddenly unloading stuff seemed to confirm my hypothesis that we can become addicted to materialism. Millions of people are coming to the same conclusion. And some have shed a hell of a lot.

In 2010, an Austrian businessman named Karl Rabeder decided to give away his entire fortune, estimated at almost $5 million. He announced he was getting rid of his villa in the Alps, his country house, and his planes, antiques, and luxury cars. He told the *Daily Telegraph*, "For a long time I believed that more wealth and luxury automatically meant more happiness. I come from a very poor family, where the rules were to work more to achieve more material things, and I applied this for many years." But, said Karl, an inner voice finally began to speak up. "More and more I heard the words: 'Stop what you are doing now—all this luxury and consumerism—and start your real life.' I had the feeling I was working as a slave for things that I did not wish for or need. I have the feeling there are a lot of people doing the same thing . . . Money is counterproductive—it prevents happiness to come." Karl said his plan was to give all his millions to charities in Latin America and live in a tiny hut in the mountains. "My idea is to have nothing left. Absolutely nothing," was how Karl summed up his plan.[1]

Now, for us non-multimillionaires, that sounds a tad eccentric. Do we really have to give up *all* of our possessions to have a more profound, more meaningful life experience? Heck no. Just like food, we need a certain amount of material possessions to live comfortably and function effectively in an increasingly complicated world. Here's the really important question:

When Does Our Consumption of Material Goods Cross a Line into Addiction?

The answer is: when we are consuming material goods for the wrong reasons, not because we really need those items but because we're scrambling to fill a void. Here's a common story: an unhappily married woman shops compulsively, spending money she doesn't have on designer shoes and handbags to escape the sadness she feels at home. Although she's a well-paid executive, her salary can't keep up with her cravings. She's put her family deeply in debt. Her husband worries over whether she has secret credit cards with even more debt he doesn't know about. Her young daughter complains that she doesn't spend enough time with her. The woman can't quit her job because she's got a flood of bills coming in every month. Yet whatever free time she has is spent buying more stuff. She is trapped in a vortex of addictive consumption and sees no way out.

We amass stuff to distract ourselves from painful, unpleasant feelings and inconvenient truths that would otherwise rise to the surface. We are also consuming for the wrong reasons when we buy something to give us status, in order to erase our feelings of insecurity. That's called *positional consumption,* because we hope it improves our position compared to someone else. Overconsumption is just like an addiction to drugs: we overconsume to escape, comfort ourselves, and numb ourselves. If you want to know if you're consuming addictively, you may want to answer these questions:

- Do you ever feel remorse after buying/consuming something? When you've bought a car/boat/time share/club membership/clothes/furniture/appliances, have you experienced an initial rush that was followed by nervousness, second guessing, and/or guilt?
- Do your shopping sprees threaten your (or your family's) financial security?
- Do you consume/shop to escape from worry or to erase a case of the blues?
- Do you fantasize that one specific purchase or material thing will make your life complete?
- Do you purchase things that you think will make you appear important and/or rich?
- Do you buy things hoping that they will impress other people?
- Do you buy things and then later wonder about the wisdom of the purchase?
- Do you covet things your friends and neighbors possess?

If you answered yes to more than a couple of these questions, you may well be consuming addictively, at least sometimes. Most of us are.

"The way that our culture is set up requires people to believe that it's important to work hard, to make a lot of money, in order to have a lot of possessions or to make more money. That's what keeps the wheels of consumer capitalism going. Materialism and high levels of consumption and shopping in some ways are a socially acceptable kind of addiction."

—Tim Kasser, author of The High Price of Materialism

America Is Using Materialism to Escape

This overconsumption of material goods is one of our most ingrained social contagions. Our entire culture has become premised on the notion of acquiring. It's the litmus test of whether you are a card-carrying citizen. Think of a band of hippies in the sixties living in a commune where it was *de rigueur* to drop acid. If you refused, you weren't really part of the cult and might be shunned or viewed with suspicion. Today, all of us are members of *the cult of consumerism.* That's why we call ourselves consumers.

Bucking the consumer mentality, becoming a free thinker and achieving emotional sobriety from overconsumption requires taking yourself out of that cult at the risk of being shunned or ridiculed! If there's one thing we know about addicts, they really don't like to use their drug with *sober* people staring at them. It puts their desperation to escape into sharp relief and brings up shame over the toxic behaviors in which they are drowning. That's why alcoholics at a party will often push cocktails on other guests. The addict feels his or her addictive behavior will be less noticeable if everybody's doing it. That's why your family, friends, and neighbors may push you to consume, even when you don't want to.

Pressure to conform to the consumer culture can be felt when a neighbor brags to you about their new purchase: "I don't know how I functioned without this self-cleaning oven" . . . or feigns shock when they learn you have failed to purchase a certain hot, new must-have: "I can't believe you don't have high def!" The unspoken message is "get with the program and buy this or you'll become a second-class citizen." Sometimes questionable consumer trends will come disguised as righteous concern for family: "I needed this SUV. I've got kids." Even though there's nothing inherently better for your family about an SUV except more space. The tradeoff is that SUVs are gas guzzlers, which negatively impacts the environment, which presumably should be preserved for the very benefit of those children sitting in the SUV. Are you really protecting your kids by buying an SUV, or are you an addict using your family as a justification for getting something you crave because you're swept up in a cultural contagion?

"We are being promised by a techno consumer culture that if we only take in more then we could be more 'ourselves.' And in the very process of pouring in more goods, more information, we are being depleted of ourselves."

—*Eugene Halton, author of* The Great Brain Suck

You Need That? Really? Seriously?

While buying something that you *actually need* is not addictive shopping, the culture has played a shell game with us, creating all manner of artificial *needs* that are really not needs at all. You can make a reasonable argument for *needing* a toaster, but do you really need a high-tech coffee maker that spits out a small, disposable, plastic coffee-grain container after every single cup it brews, a container that's extremely hard to recycle because it's filled with wet, used coffee grains? These environmentally insensitive individual-cup coffee makers are now popping up in homes and offices everywhere.

Birthdays, baby showers, weddings, the ever-growing number of holidays, and all other special occasions are opportunities to enforce the rules of the cult. You *need* to get a wedding gift! You *need* to send a card on Mother's Day. You *need* to buy everyone you know some kind of present for Christmas or Hanukah. NO, YOU DON'T! Not if you don't listen to the cult. There are many other ways to say "I love you." In fact, you can just *say*, "I love you" and mean it. You can make a donation to a charity in someone's name. You can re-gift things you've been given but can't use. I have a friend who keeps a big box where she puts all the stuff she can no longer use. She carefully matches up these items with the needs of her friends and is always bearing gifts, albeit previously owned ones. Now I'm starting to do it too. It's a fun way to get rid of clutter.

The First Step Toward Freedom from Any Addiction Is to Admit You Have It

We simply cannot continue living the way we are without destroying our physical world. But to change, we must first acknowledge the truth: America is addicted to stuff. The mob psychosis that demands material gifts for all these occasions is wreaking havoc on our finances and on the environment. The wrapping paper alone is an ecological disaster, with Americans piling up 4 million tons of waste every year just from wrapping paper and holiday shopping bags. Four million tons![2] That's a lot of forests destroyed. For what? Something you look at for five seconds before

ripping it away? In fact, paper products are the second most frequently purchased packaged goods found in American homes, right
after bread and other baked goods.[3] With the exception of toilet
paper, lots of those paper goods are totally unnecessary. Gee, what
did people do before they had paper towels? A simple switch to
dishrags would save forests and dramatically reduce pollution from
manufacturing sources. Absent that, a simple switch to recycled
paper towels would do wonders. The recycled paper company Seventh Generation lays it out right on its paper towel wrapper, noting,
"If every household in the U.S. replaced just one roll of 120 ct. virgin
fiber paper towels with a 100% recycled one, we could save:

- 933,000 trees
- 2.4 million cubic feet of landfill space, equal to
  3,700 full garbage trucks
- 350 million gallons of water, a year's supply for
  2,700 families of four
- and avoid 59,600 tons of emissions."[4]

We all know the truth in our bones. We Americans are using way
more than our fair share of the world's finite resources. The United States
accounts for about 5 percent of the world's population yet accounts for
one-third of global consumption![5] We're all screaming statistics at each
other, and yet the freight train of overconsumption is only accelerating.
That's because addiction does not respond to rational argument.

"Addiction does not have to be a physical drug. Drugs provide
biochemical indoctrination. If you shoot heroin, you will become
biochemically indoctrinated and habituated to it. That's on everybody's radar. What's off the radar is electrochemical indoctrination. When you see ads, they jolt your adrenaline. They change
you physiologically. They are intended to do that. They create

physiological habits. When you watch 3,500 ads every day—with a large percentage telling you that you are inadequate until you get the commodity—that's bound to have an effect on people."

*—Eugene Halton, Ph.D., professor of sociology
at the University of Notre Dame*

Drowning in Consumer Debris

American overconsumption is a mass addiction. The average household contains more televisions than human beings. The United States has more cars than drivers. Every year we spend more than $22 billion on health clubs and health equipment. But on any given day, three-quarters of us are doing no exercise at all.[6] *Zip!* It feels good to plunk down our credit card for a health club membership. We do so fantasizing about how buffed we're going to get and how attractive we'll look to others. Unfortunately, fantasizing doesn't burn a whole lot of calories. How many of us have gym memberships that we never use? Actually working out is a lot sweatier than fantasizing about it or paying for the privilege. And to work out, we'd actually have to look in the mirror and see the disturbing "before" picture of how we look now!

Instead of Running, Dancing, Swimming, or Singing, We're . . . Hoarding!

If you find yourself having difficulty deciding what's valuable and what's not or if you feel irrational attachment to material items, you may be on the path to a deeper manifestation of the compulsion to collect called hoarding. Two million of us are compulsive hoarders.[7] The phenomenon has even inspired two disturbing reality TV shows: *Hoarders* and *Hoarding: Buried Alive.*[8] The shows follow people who fill their homes with mountains of debris because they are completely traumatized by the thought of throwing anything out. This can even include dirty diapers, rotten food, and dead animals. Ironically, a common reason offered by hoarders to keep an object is its sentimental family value. But their hoarding is precisely what keeps their families alienated. Relatives refuse to visit because a hoarder's home is generally filled with such squalor it's nauseating and unsafe. Many hoarders admit to being powerless over the urge to buy. They may have closets stuffed with clothes they've never worn, but still can't resist picking up a new sweater at a department-store sale. Eventually, they begin to drown in junk.

In Las Vegas, a compulsive hoarder was dead for four months before her husband finally discovered her body under piles of debris in their home. Her clutter was so intense that even search dogs (who had worked Ground Zero and Hurricane Katrina) had failed to sniff her out.[9]

Materialism Is an Expensive Habit!

The average rate of personal savings falls short of what most people need to feel secure. Millions of households actually spend more than their after-tax income.[10] No wonder we're stressed out. Total U.S. consumer debt is in the staggering trillions of dollars. Many Americans are in a serious debt trap, with credit cards, home equity lines, and home mortgages eating up an increasing slice of their income. They've overspent to such an extent that they're reduced to treading water financially, working just to keep up with their monthly interest payments. The banks encouraged a lot of this debt by *enabling* people to pretend they were wealthy through an ever-more-imaginative rollout of credit vehicles. Take second mortgages. Taking out a second mortgage on your home used to be a sign of financial desperation. But the banks renamed second mortgages "home equity loans" and encouraged Americans to raid and pillage their own castles. As one bank ad proclaimed, "There's got to be at least $25,000 hidden in your house. We can help you find it." Home equity loans became a social contagion![11] Of course, when the real-estate bubble hit, those with two mortgages found themselves in double trouble, much more likely to be upside down on their house. Here's the added danger of social contagions. They make self-destructive behavior like massive personal debt socially acceptable. That, in turn, gives people a false sense of security. But there is no safety in numbers. If I'm thundering toward a sharp cliff, I may feel safer if I'm part of a huge herd doing the same thing. But in reality, it simply means we're all going to die. After the real-estate bubble burst, the cult of consumerism started feeling more like the 1970s killer cult of Jim Jones.

Most addicts don't ponder the cost or consequences of their habit. Getting their next fix is always priority number one, so very few addicts seriously plan for the future. Most Americans live in complete denial about how much they will need to live decently in retirement. The Motley Fool puts it this way: "Let's say you're retiring in thirty years, and you want to live off the equivalent of $50,000 a year in today's dollars. By then, that $50,000 will need to be $150,000 thanks to inflation, and if that amount is 4 percent of your savings (the guideline espoused by the Fool's *Rule Your Retirement* service), your total retirement kitty will have to total $3.75 million."[12] Good luck with that.

Meanwhile, as we fail to plan for our retirement, the pushers of products have developed a growing body of scientific research centered on understanding why people buy for all sorts of irrational and unconscious reasons. It's all part of a master plan to figure out new ways to get us to buy even more. In the United States alone, market research is a $12 billion a year industry.[13] Martin Lindstrom, the author of the revealing book *Buyology* is a global branding expert and a leader in the field of neuromarketing. Using cutting-edge brain-scanning instruments, he has studied the brainwaves of thousands of volunteers as they're shown ads, commercials, logos, and products.[14] He writes that his research "revealed the hidden truths behind how branding and marketing messages work on the human brain, how our truest selves react to stimuli at a level far deeper than conscious thought, and how our unconscious minds control our behavior (usually the opposite of how we *think* we behave)."[15]

"The government is so often focused on economic growth as the 'be all' and 'end all' of its aims. And of course economic growth relies about 70 percent on consumption in a nation like ours. You can see it in the thousands of commercial impressions that children and adults are exposed to every day—all of which have the same underlying message: buy something and your life will be better."

—Tim Kasser, professor and chair of psychology at Knox College

---

Often the reasons for a purchase have little to do with practicality and rational need and much more to do with deep-seated, even primal desires for social acceptance, sex, and status. Lindstrom describes one study where a car maker showed volunteers various images of automobiles and observed, ". . . just as male peacocks attract female mates with the iridescence of their back feathers, the males in this study subconsciously sought to attract the opposite sex with the low-rising, engine-revving, chrome pizzazz of the sports car."[16]

Unlike peacocks, human beings are supposed to be able to manage their instincts and impulses. Addiction is what happens when our instincts betray us. When we get an urge to buy something, it often feels *urgent*, like an instinctual desire such as an itch we need to scratch. In fact, our instinctive responses are often being artificially triggered by subliminal signals sent to our subconscious that manipulate us into associating the product with the fulfillment of a primal urge, like sex. But it's all a mirage. An expensive men's watch doesn't make a man more virile or powerful. And a fur coat—no matter what the price—is a cruel obscenity that certainly doesn't make a woman look sexier. It makes her look barbaric.

When hit with a seemingly uncontrollable urge to buy, it's interesting to notice what fantasies are coming up in one's mind in relation to the product. Are you visualizing yourself with the product in a grandiose way, admired by others? Such fantasies would be a tipoff that you're seeking something this inanimate product will never be able to deliver.

"Part of this process of building our consumption culture, is to transform citizens into consumers. A consumer is a much smaller thing than a citizen. If you can get people to stop realizing that they have public lives that they can live in their communities and neighborhoods, if you get them to narrow down to think of themselves as just a consumer, then you get them hooked on this stimulus response model and the idea that they are only going to complete themselves through further purchasing."

—Gene Halton, Ph.D., professor of sociology
at the University of Notre Dame

We know addictive behavior gets worse over time. That's true with booze and it's true with stuff. The United States and Europe are hoarding more and more of the world's resources. The wealthiest 20 percent of the world accounts for three-quarters of total private consumption. The poorest fifth of the world accounts for barely a bleep.[17] I'm talking about stuff: clothes, shoes, cars, houses, dvds, books, furniture, toys, electronics, housewares, plastic bottles, and so on. Less than a quarter of the world's humans gobble up three-quarters of the world's stuff! It's time we all ask ourselves, *Am I part of that "20 percent" in the massive overconsumption range?*

In the national bestseller *Why We Buy*, retail guru Paco Underhill—whose clients have included some of the biggest brand names in the world—explains why corporations hire him to videotape shoppers and analyze their buying habits: "If we went into stores only when we needed to buy something, and if once there we bought only what we needed, the economy would collapse—boom. Fortunately, the economic party that started the second half of the twentieth century has fostered more shopping than anyone would have predicted, more shopping than has ever taken place anywhere at any time. You almost have to make an effort to avoid shopping today."[18] That's the understatement of the century!

While Underhill doesn't see this overconsumption epidemic in the sinister light I do, he does issue a fascinating warning: "Every expert agrees, we are now dangerously over-retailed—too much is for sale, through too many outlets. The economy even at its strongest can't keep up with retailing's growth. Judging from birthrates, we're generating stores a lot faster than we're producing new shoppers."[19]

Leave it to a retail guru to describe a fatal flaw in our consumer culture. Our entire economy is teetering on a house of cards. And his description dovetails perfectly with the dynamics of addiction. Addiction is always about *too much*! An alcoholic drinks *too much*! A food addict eats *too much!* A gambling addict gambles *too much*! A shopaholic shops *too much*! A culture addicted to consumption *produces too much* for us to consume and offers too many ways for us to consume it! We have too many stores, too many outlets, too many malls, too many boutiques, too many department stores. We're constantly concocting products that claim to be "new and improved" to manipulate status- and novelty-obsessed consumers into buying that too. It's all *too much*!

In fact, we now have so much unnecessary stuff that self-storage has become a huge industry! Hideously ugly self-storage facilities are popping up all over the country like pimples as people store all the crap that they never should have bought in the first place and for which they have no room. The truth is that absent food, toothpaste, shampoo, electricity, Internet/cell phone connectivity, and gas, most of us could go for years without actually *needing* to buy much of anything. In fact, there is a new philosophy whimsically dubbed "Enoughism."[20] The concept is that at a certain point consumers actually own everything they need and buying anything more starts to make their lives worse, not better. Like any addiction, materialism starts out as fun and then crosses a line into fun with problems and, finally, steers us into misery.

The Big Consumer Economy Con Game

We are constantly being told that economic growth is essential to our economic well-being. Since American consumers account for two-thirds of domestic economic activity, that means average Americans are being told they *need* to keep spending for our society's very survival. Everything depends on our going shopping! But here's why it's all a big con game at your expense. The capital being generated isn't being distributed to the average American. The capital being generated by all this unnecessary shopping is increasingly being collected by a tiny percentage of the population.

More and more wealth is being concentrated in the hands of fewer and fewer people. For decades, CEOs have been getting mind-boggling raises, even as they've presided over massive layoffs. How's your standard of living improved by comparison? Unless you're at the top of the income ladder, chances are your answer is "not much."

The vast majority of taxpayers have seen their incomes remain nearly flat for the last three decades. But income for the top 0.01 percent shot heavenward by almost 1,000 percent! [21] I'm going to think about *that* the next time I'm being swayed to buy some gizmo I don't really need.

Our Addiction to Materialism Is Creating Wealth Disparity

The unspoken promise of this so-called capitalism is that we too could, one day, become billionaires. Hey, it could happen. We could win the lottery several times in a row. But what's the chance of that happening? Slim to none. Nevertheless, we consumers—brain-washed and addicted—march in lockstep, proudly defending capitalism, even though it's not really capitalism anymore. And it's certainly not making most of us rich.

Faux Capitalism

Hey, I enjoyed those Ayn Rand books as much as anybody. I'd love to spend a night tooling around town with John Galt or Howard Roark, Rand's fictional heroes who personify the capitalistic ethos. But I hate to break it to you . . . we no longer live in a capitalistic society. The dictionary definition of capitalism is "An economic system based on a free market, open competition, profit motive and private ownership of the means of production." But today, the so-called "free market" is hardly free! It's ironic that anyone who challenges today's economic system is accused of being a socialist, because what we have today is actually *corporate socialism*. Giant for-profit corporations consistently get unfair advantages and subsidies from government, undermining the whole concept of open competition.

Big Business Controls Our Government

Capitalism's sacred law of supply and demand has been perverted by our morally bankrupt political culture. Entrenched, corrupt government bureaucrats consistently give rapacious corporate behemoths an unfair advantage over small, local, progressive, ecologically minded and ethically aware private enterprises. Big business has its thumb on the scale.

Corporate interests dominate most government agencies, effectively reducing them to ethical wastelands. In her must-read book, *The Story of Stuff,* Annie Leonard writes, "In the United States there are about 900 advisory committees that provide peer review of scientific research, develop policy recommendations . . . and serve other functions to support good governance. These committees are so active in providing advice to Congress, federal agencies, and the President that they are sometimes referred to as the 'fifth arm of government.' Federal law requires that these independent committees have members who represent a balanced diversity of views and who are free from conflicts of interests . . . however, industry influence continues to dominate these committees."[23]

In other words, these powerful committees are loaded with businesspeople who stand to make their industries bigger profits by influencing the committee's recommendations. Government agencies also have been known to base their decisions on studies funded by biased parties like industry trade groups.

> "These are very good ways to addict people: to create a culture of people who have been smothered before they can even develop through a combination of technology, media, and consumption dictates. Is that good for growth? It probably is. But is it good for the growth of the individuals involved? No."
>
> —*Eugene Halton, author of* The Great Brain Suck

Addicted to Growth

Corporate greed is the other side of the overconsumption coin. Why are we being pressured to buy so much stuff? Because America's corporate culture is addicted to constant revenue growth! America's CEOs are hooked on showing ever-increasing profits, quarter by quarter, to meet or beat analysts' expectations. As ponzi schemer Bernie Madoff proved, you can't profit unwaveringly without taking ethical shortcuts. And the accessory to corporate crime is usually the U.S. government. We have a fox-guarding-the-henhouse problem in almost every agency of government, from the USDA to the FDA to the Interior Department. The U.S. government looks the other way while corporate giants decimate taxpayer-owned public lands and natural resources, risking the safety and health of our citizens. Take big oil.

Who could ever forget that terrible day in the spring of 2010 when oil started spilling into the Gulf of Mexico? The slow-moving apocalypse killed eleven workers, laid waste to large swaths of the Gulf of Mexico, and threatened countless species of wildlife and vast stretches of shoreline. Soon, America learned that the oil company had decided several days before the deadly rig explosion to choose a type of casing for the well that it knew was the riskier of the two options. Why? For one thing, it was cheaper. In the oil company's own documents, the strategy was described as "best economic case."[24]

Where were the federal inspectors who are charged with looking out for our interests, given that the drilling was occurring on public property? God only knows. Perhaps engaged in a beer-pong contest. As the devastation mounted, a government report revealed that federal inspectors overseeing oil drilling in the Gulf of Mexico regularly chowed down on free meals and took tickets to sporting events from the very companies they monitored. The report said some of the government inspectors even let oil company workers fill out their inspection forms in pencil, which the inspectors simply copied over in ink before submitting them. One inspector admitted, "Everyone has gotten some sort of gift . . ." from the companies they were supposed to be scrutinizing.[25]

This should have come as no surprise. About two years before this disaster, while Congress was debating the wisdom of expanding oil drilling in coastal waters owned by taxpayers, a scandal erupted over sex and drug use within the Interior Department agency that oversees oil drilling. Reports detailed "a culture of substance abuse and promiscuity" where government officials "frequently consumed alcohol at industry functions, had used cocaine and marijuana, and had sexual relationships with oil and gas company representatives."[26] So when we talk about government being in bed with big oil, we're not exaggerating.

Hooked and Cooked on Oil

Big oil is the big elephant in the room when it comes to overconsumption. It's not just gas. It's plastic. Plastic cups, plastic water bottles, plastic forks and knives, plastic bags . . . they are all made

from petrochemicals! Oil—petroleum—is a key ingredient in petrochemicals![27] The next time we casually toss away a plastic water bottle we should pause to think of the catastrophic Gulf oil spill. If we
really look hard into those oily waters, we just might see our own
reflection.

Most of the plastic we use is not biodegradable. Some plastics
become toxic when burned. Plastic bags from the supermarket take
1,000 years to degrade. But, still, we thoughtlessly accept them
because, oops, we forgot to bring that reusable bag from home. A
heroin junkie's home is rarely neat. Similarly, our cultural addictions
are making for a trashy nation and a filthy world. In the Pacific
Ocean, somewhere between California and Hawaii, there's a cluster of
trash that's at least twice the size of Texas. Millions of tons of plastic
wind up in oceans every year.[28]

Addictive behavior invariably leads to moral degeneracy, and cultural addictions are no exception. While we've become a nation of
oil junkies, mired in our own oil-based trash, our oil pushers behave
like mob bosses, bullying and breaking anyone who stands in their
way. And, like a mob boss, an oil-industry official who was on the
rig the day of the Gulf oil rig explosion took the Fifth, refusing to
testify at an investigative hearing for fear of incriminating himself.
In my mind, the Gulf oil spill marked a turning point and a tipping
point. After decades of living in denial, we Americans were finally
forced to stare at the consequences of our consumer lifestyle. The oil
slick became a metaphor for everything wrong with our materialistic culture. It was as if the whole country was being dragged into an
intervention.

But what's the alternative to our messed-up system? Must we
really choose between unsustainable economic growth that's destroying our environment or the collapse of our entire economy and the

prospect of another Great Depression? Perhaps it is time to ask, What's behind door number three?

"All the data show that increased economic growth in the United States over the last 50 years has not promoted higher levels of well-being among the citizens."

—*Tim Kasser, author of* The High Price of Materialism

There Is Another Way

There are really two challenges here. One is micro, one is macro. One is what we, as individuals, can do to break our overconsumption habit. The other is what society and its institutions—including government—must do to revamp our economic systems so they value something beyond just economic growth, which is simply not ecologically sustainable.

A growing chorus of environmentally minded economists are demanding that we, as a culture and an economy, stop measuring ourselves by GDP (gross domestic product), which is the market value of all the goods and services made in the United States every year. GDP is often associated with the standard of living.

There is now a new movement to come up with a less materialistic measuring stick to assess the nation's well-being. GNH or *Gross National Happiness* is a concept that has sprung up as a more holistic, more spiritual measure of how we, as in *We the People*, are faring. It seeks to measure not just how many *goods* we're churning out but how *good* we feel. It would assign values to intangibles like the social and psychological contentedness of citizens and the health of our environment. Supporters describe this new outlook as "measuring what matters."

In the excellent book *Prosperity Without Growth*, Tim Jackson argues that we need to redefine prosperity, noting "Unraveling the culture—and changing the social logic—of consumerism will require the kind of sustained and systematic effort it took to put it in place to start with. Crucially though, this effort clearly won't succeed as a purely punitive endeavor. Offering people viable alternatives to the consumer way of life is vital. Progress depends on building up capabilities for people to flourish in less materialistic ways."[29]

You have to offer a better alternative is a fundamental truth of addiction. You don't just stop drinking. You have to replace alcohol with something else that will give you pleasure in a different way, a sober way. Let's examine sober pleasure versus addictive pleasure. Addictive pleasure creates a rush, a high, and later a crash. For example, there's the rush of buying something expensive and then the crash of getting the credit card bill. Sober pleasure is more incremental and stretched out. Walking on the beach, visiting a museum, or volunteering for a charity doesn't provide the same rush, but neither does it wallop you with a crash.

In order to break our addiction to materialism, we need to cultivate more nonmaterial pleasures. What are some of the nonmaterial things we value?

- We value our time.
- We value our experience of nature.
- We value our sense of spiritual well-being,
  which comes from being of service to others.

We need to start giving currency to these intangibles, so they can be measured and traded on the open market.

Let's address time. If our culture valued time more, we could create a system that would give people more free time, more vacation time, more time to work from home. Perhaps a four-day work week, more part-time jobs, more staggered commuting hours, more opportunities to work from home, and more telecommuting. With conference calling, Skype, and Internet interconnectivity, plenty of people who endure grueling commutes could instead work from home. This would automatically reduce our gas consumption and our total carbon footprint. Spreading out the workload would allow us to employ more people, thereby reducing the fear of widespread unemployment due to lower GDP. Tax breaks could encourage corporations to embrace flextime and part-time strategies.

Let's tackle nature. A big part of our dilemma is that we have not assigned a negative value to the destruction of our ecosystem in the calculations we make to assess the nation's economic well-being. We need to hold industry much more accountable for environmental wreckage, exploitation, and cruelty.

One innovate way to do that would be to assign "rights" to certain entities in our world which have heretofore been denied them. If natural entities, like bodies of water, such as the Gulf of Mexico, were assigned "natural rights," there would be a total prohibition on the kind of disastrous pollution that is now occurring. It simply would not be allowed because it would be a violation of its natural rights. We'd be forced to come up with alternatives to gas and oil-based plastics. Innovative, ecologically minded entrepreneurs could devise such alternatives, spurring a new wave of ecologically minded economic development. In fact, there are already completely biodegradable plant-based water bottles, but—thus far—there has been no incentive for major water bottle manufacturers to switch to them. This new "rights" system would provide such an incentive.

Similarly, if we assigned natural entities, such as forests, natural rights, we would drastically limit the amount of trees used for paper products. Tough, new criteria would be established to justify the destruction of a tree, which would make wanton use of virgin wood economically unfeasible, forcing paper companies to switch to recycled paper en masse. If *Seventh Generation* can do it, why can't all the other companies? The answer is: they can. They just won't do it until they're pushed, either by a new economic system or by consumer demand.

Similarly, there are many products that are made from animal skins and parts for which there are compassionate alternatives. If we formally recognized that the millions of animals raised and killed for fashion in America every year had "inalienable rights" to humane treatment, it would effectively put the fur industry out of business. Ditto for many of the food products we consume. The elimination of massive industrial farms would reduce our carbon footprint enormously as meat production is the single biggest cause of global warming, far beyond transportation, according to an in-depth United Nations study. The assignment of such rights would require giving cows, pigs, sheep, chickens, and other farm animals room to move, access to the outdoors, and opportunities to socialize. This would make meat more expensive, which would encourage people to eat differently and incorporate more varieties of vegetables, grains, and legumes into their diet. Different kinds of private enterprises would spring up to meet these new demands. Food cooperatives would flourish. Fast food would decline and perhaps cease to exist. Obesity would plummet. The health of Americans would improve. Our GNH (gross national happiness) would skyrocket.

Some might call this compassionate capitalism. While many of the suggested environmental reforms, like cap and trade, are extraordinarily complex, the assignment of rights to animals and nature is an extraordinarily simple way to achieve the same results. "Natural rights" could be assigned to land, water, air, domestic farm animals, and wild animals. That would instantly criminalize much of the rapacious destruction of the environment occurring by private industry today. For those who say this would wreak economic havoc, well . . . that's what critics said about the elimination of slavery too.

Beyond that, America needs to start being of service to the rest of humanity, making goods that people around the world desperately need, like systems to produce drinkable water, promote birth control, and improve sanitation. The list is long. It's incomprehensible that we Americans are drowning in material items while a good percentage of the world's population barely owns a toothbrush. At least 3 billion people—almost half the world's population—live on less than $2.50 a day. [30] It's true that Third World consumers don't have much to spend. But that's where recovery principles come in. We, in the developed world, need to make *amends* for the destruction we have wrought on so many developing countries. We need to start producing not to profit, but to satisfy real, pressing needs of those half a world away. Ironically, this may boost our Gross National Happiness like nothing else.

Chapter Two
THE PHARMERS: Addicted to Pharmaceuticals
-- -- -- -- -- -- -- -- -- -- --

Every so often we wake up with no clue that this will become one of those days to remember. It's June 25, 2009. I am in gloriously sunny Puerto Rico, and it's the first time I have taken any time off since I started my HLN TV show *Issues* eight months earlier. The National Association of Hispanic Journalists is having its yearly convention in San Juan. The palm trees are dancing to a fragrant tropical breeze as recognizable TV hosts and reporters from all over the country chat one another up in the open-air lobby of a gorgeous oceanfront hotel. Suddenly, a weird energy starts to ripple through the crowd. Heads dip down toward their BlackBerrys. My cell phone rings. It's my show's senior booker.

"Jane, hi, sorry to interrupt your vacation but," she paused ominously, " . . . we think Michael Jackson is dead."

I am staring at the gorgeous Caribbean sea, but my mind is suddenly oceans away. A few miles inland from the Pacific Ocean, in Los Angeles, Michael Jackson has been transported to a hospital. He is not breathing and is soon pronounced dead. His family believes he was dead on arrival and are convinced he was murdered.[1]

Almost immediately, my friends start texting me: "Y R U in PR? MJ's DEAD!!!" I take it personally for a moment. "I'M NOT A PSYCHIC!!" is my irritated reply. This is the biggest celebrity news to break since my show started, and I'm stranded on an island thousands of miles away from this monumental story. Since I was one of a small cluster of reporters in the courtroom for the entire Michael Jackson molestation trial, I'm particularly associated with all things Jackson. Talk about bad timing! My frustration meter is peaking, but I force myself to let it go with a shrug because I'm totally powerless over this predicament.

Fortunately for me, this is a story with . . . as they say . . . legs.

In the coming days, the world would learn about the King of Pop's addiction to his "milk." That was Jackson's nickname for the powerful surgical knockout drug propofol, which is only supposed to be used in hospital settings to put patients under for surgery. Doctors have jokingly called the white liquid "milk of amnesia" for its ability to almost instantly render a person completely unconscious. It would turn out that Michael was using propofol as a sleep aid to get some serious naptime in as he prepared for his make-or-break comeback tour ironically entitled "This Is It." Propofol would literally knock him out in a second or two, guaranteeing the superstar at least a few hours' respite from his chronic insomnia.

Michael Jackson had an in-house physician, Dr. Conrad Murray, who would later be charged with involuntary manslaughter for his actions in the hours leading up to Jackson's death. Cops say the doctor admitted to giving Jackson a head-spinning cocktail of drugs over the course of just a few hours. The list included the sedatives Valium, lorazepam (Ativan), and midazolam (Versed), plus the painkiller lidocaine, topped off with propofol (Diprivan).[2]

While the circumstances of Michael Jackson's death may have seemed shocking, they shouldn't have surprised anyone. A couple of years before his death, Michael Jackson had been sued after racking up a $100,000 tab at a Beverly Hills pharmacy.[3] Famous friends, from Uri Geller to Deepak Chopra, were extremely concerned about the star: Chopra refused him painkillers, and Gellar warned Jackson he was going to die if he continued to abuse drugs.[4] But here's the key fact—not a single drug mentioned in connection with Michael Jackson's death is an illegal drug. They were all *legal* prescription drugs being inappropriately prescribed and then abused by perhaps the world's most famous, and arguably, most talented pill popper.

Falling Stars

Michael Jackson has plenty of competition. The list of celebrities who have overdosed on legal prescription drugs is long and growing fast. Heath Ledger overdosed in his fashionable Manhattan loft on a combination of oxycodone, hydrocodone, diazepam, alprazolam, temazepam, and doxylamine, otherwise known as the painkillers OxyContin and Vicodin, the antianxiety drugs Valium and Xanax, and the sleep aids Restoril and Unisom.[5] Again, all perfectly legal . . . and all potentially deadly when combined and otherwise misused. Anna Nicole Smith had a head-spinning array of legal prescription drugs in her system when she died in a Florida hotel room. Lexapro, Zoloft, Cipro, Klonopin, Valium, Ativan, Robaxin, and the powerful sleep aid chloral hydrate were found in her system. Reports claimed that toward the end, Anna Nicole was slugging chloral hydrate right out of the bottle.[6]

Shop to Pop Till You Drop

We've all heard about secretly addicted patients who go from doctor to doctor, claiming all sorts of ailments, from back pain to migraines, convincing each physician to prescribe painkillers before moving on to the next M.D. Many of these patients will also go into psychological therapy to squeeze antianxiety meds and antidepressants out of their psychiatrists. The various doctors don't know about each other and have no idea (or pretend to have no idea) that their patient is shopping around for as many drugs as he or she can get. The fact is, if someone is strung out on pills, it eventually becomes rather obvious. Their eyes are glassy, and they're often twitchy and scattered. Many doctors prefer not to notice and collect their fees rather than risk an uncomfortable confrontation with a patient demanding drugs, who will always ferociously insist it's to relieve exquisite pain. Drug addicts, in their desperation to score, can be very persuasive.

Eighties' TV and movie star Corey Haim may well become the poster child for doctor shopping. In March 2010, the *Lost Boys* actor collapsed and died in his mother's Los Angeles apartment, at the age of thirty-eight. While he had very bad chest congestion, many in Hollywood immediately suspected an overdose. For decades, Corey had been an incorrigible drug addict. He once described himself on *Larry King Live* as a "chronic relapser." The prescription-pill habit got so bad that he became almost destitute.

Corey's agent insisted that, when he took Corey on as a client about a year and a half before his death, he did it on the condition that Corey get clean. His agent insisted to me "live" on *Issues* that Corey had cleaned up his act. The agent was convinced Corey didn't die of a drug overdose, although he added Corey might have had a bad reaction to medications his addiction specialist was giving him. Wait! A doctor was giving Corey Haim drugs in order to get him off drugs? That makes no sense to me. Some drug addicts, when they first get sober, are so riddled with drugs they need to be gradually weaned off so they don't go into convulsions or worse. But that process should never take a year and a half. If the agent had insisted a year and a half earlier that Corey get clean, then Corey should not have been taking *any* drugs, period!

Sobriety means the absence of *all* mood-altering drugs with the rare exception of an absolute medical necessity, and then for only as long as absolutely medically necessary. Sobriety does not mean giving the addict less-potent drugs. That's called "managing" your addiction, and it's almost always guaranteed to fail because an addict is precisely someone who cannot practice moderation. Most people seem to understand this concept when it comes to alcohol, but sometimes get confused when it comes to prescription pills because they're "medicine." Just as a drunk cannot have a sip of alcohol without triggering a craving that can result in a major binge, so a pill head cannot take any mood-altering pills because even half a pill can provoke a powerful craving for a lot more of the same. Even half a pill puts addicts *into their disease*, physically, emotionally, and psychologically. Still, addicts often manage to use the "I'm weaning myself off" excuse to score more drugs.

"It's not a Hollywood issue. It's a country-wide issue that only gets talked about when the rich and famous die."

–Howard Samuels, Psy.D., licensed clinical psychologist,
founder, and CEO of the Hills Treatment Center in Los Angeles

---

The controversy over Corey's death dominated the headlines. As we all waited for the inevitably slow toxicology report to come back, more and more reports surfaced that Corey was still up to his old tricks. California's then–attorney general Jerry Brown announced that Corey Haim's name had popped up on a fraudulently obtained prescription for the powerful drug OxyContin, which is sometimes referred to as "Hillbilly Heroin."[7] The phony prescription scheme was linked to a massive illegal prescription drug ring operating out of Southern California. Brown said this ring would steal legitimate doctors' identities and use that information to print up phony prescription pads. Prescription pads are like cash; they're a currency unto themselves. The counterfeit prescriptions were then sold to drug abusers and street pushers, who would go to drugstore after drugstore to get massive quantities of pills.

Brown added that Corey was also going to legitimate doctors and obtaining prescriptions from them. Haim's name came up on multiple prescriptions in the state's system. "He had dozens of doctors, many, many prescriptions, using many, many pharmacies, more than a dozen," said Brown,[8] who tallied the total number of prescription pills obtained by the actor in the months before his death at more than 500. This would appear to be classic "doctor shopping."

When the coroner's conclusions were finally issued, we were told Corey Haim died of "natural" causes from pneumonia that had damaged his lungs, complicated by an enlarged heart and clogged arteries. But even though the coroner said drugs didn't kill him or contribute to his death, they did find low levels of eight different drugs in his system. The toxicology tests turned up the antidepressant fluoxetine (Prozac), the antipsychotic olanzapine, the antianxiety drug diazepam (Valium), the muscle relaxer carisoprodol, and the tranquilizer meprobamate. He was also taking a cough suppressant and an antihistamine.[9]

Additionally, the coroner's investigative report noted several bottles of prescription pills were found in Haim's name, including hydrocodone, the key ingredient in Vicodin. The narrative adds, "The decedent usually took 7 Tylenol PMs every night to help him sleep," although he did not take any on the last night of his life.

While my heart goes out to his family, that is not a profile of sobriety. As a recovering alcoholic, I can attest that everything an addict does is skewed and poisoned by the obsession to use. If I had died before I got sober, alcohol would have been a huge factor, even if I was technically sober at the moment of death. Addiction destroys your ability to take care of yourself. And that can impact everything from your grooming to your health.

These tragic cases get lots of attention, from the media and from law enforcement, because they involve famous people. But all over America, not-so-famous people are seeing their lives destroyed by prescription drugs. They're keeling over, left and right, from meds prescribed by their doctors, and nobody is doing a damn thing! This crisis is much more widespread than even the overdose statistics reflect. Tens of millions of Americans are walking, working, and driving around in an unnecessary and debilitating fog because they're high on a little pill that they got from their doctor.

Robert DuPont, a former White House drug czar who once ran the National Institute on Drug Abuse, put it bluntly: "The biggest and fastest-growing part of America's drug problem is prescription drug abuse."[10] In 2009, powerful narcotic painkillers accounted for almost 10 percent of all prescribed drugs.[11]

America's Real Drug Conspiracy

Law enforcement, the federal government, the medical community, and the pharmaceutical industry all have a vested interest in maintaining the status quo. The result is that illegal drug users and pushers, who are mostly poor and minority, are being prosecuted in huge numbers while the abusers of legal prescription drugs, who are mostly middle-class whites, are getting high with little reason to worry about being incarcerated.

> "For the upper middle class it's a lot safer to go to a doctor and get these drugs than it is to go on the street and put yourself at risk of being arrested."
>
> *—Howard Samuels, Psy.D., licensed clinical psychologist, founder, and CEO of the Hills Treatment Center*

Our nation is in the throes of a prescription drug abuse crisis of unprecedented proportions, and our myopic, jaded, and complacent criminal justice system is in see-no-evil, hear-no-evil mode!

Corey Haim was allegedly going to dozens of doctors. Did those doctors ever think to Google the star's name to see if he had a reputation for being a druggie? Had they taken this simple step, his own pronouncements about his being a chronic relapser would have popped right up. And we know Haim's name came up in the state system in connection with numerous prescriptions. In an effort to cut down on rampant prescription drug abuse, California has created a program that gives doctors and pharmacists real-time access to a patient's history of prescription drug use. More than 100 million dispensed drugs are listed in that database, and every year 60,000 doctors and pharmacists ask the right questions.[12] But clearly there are plenty of doctors who don't want to know.

Our War on Some Drugs

The truth is: America's taxpayer-funded "War on Drugs" is primarily a war on illegal drugs, like cocaine and heroin. Depending on how you estimate it, Uncle Sam spends at least $13 billion a year in the War on Drugs.[13] Some insist it's more than twice that. That's nuts! Has it put so much as a dent in the drug cartels wreaking havoc on our border? This misguided war continues even though prescription painkillers have now surpassed heroin and cocaine as the leading cause of fatal overdoses. The Centers for Disease Control (CDC) says more than 26,000 Americans overdose every year.[14] *Most* of these fatal ODs are caused by prescription drugs! Nation-wide, deaths from prescription-drug overdoses are the second-leading cause of accidental death behind car accidents. *In some states, prescription-drug overdoses are the leading cause of accidental fatalities.*[15]

But for the most part, this epidemic is being ignored. Meanwhile, addicts take advantage of the lack of scrutiny to game the system. On *Issues*, I spoke with a recovering addict who we called Nikki, not her real name. Nikki appeared in silhouette to explain how she doctor-shopped with impunity, selling some of the prescription drugs she obtained, while downing the rest to feed her own habit.

NIKKI, RECOVERING PRESCRIPTION PILL ADDICT: I went to about four different doctors at a time. After having multiple spinal surgeries, I used to keep my records with me. I would go to the doctor, and I would say, "I want to get a doctor closer to home or I want to get a doctor closer to work" . . . I had two doctors in the city, one in the sub-urbs and one in another borough.

Most of the time I would say to them, "You know, I've been on very strong medication for a very long time, and I want to wean off of some of it." So I would tell them exactly what milligram I wanted to come down to.

To have it covered by insurance, as long as the strength and milligrams was different, you could get as many prescriptions as you want for that month. So I could have four different prescriptions for OxyContin, as long as the strength was different.[16]

VELEZ-MITCHELL: That is absolutely mind-boggling. Now we're hearing the ex-fiancée say Corey Haim took forty, fifty pills (a day). How many pills were you taking at the height of this?

NIKKI: I was probably taking about that many . . . OxyContin more than anything else. Everything else was just more of a chaser. The OxyContin is what really had me to my knees.

VELEZ-MITCHELL: Why didn't the doctors pick up on it? That's what everybody wonders.

NIKKI: Well, you know, I had a valid injury. And to tell you the truth, I quote unquote, don't look like a drug addict. You know, we're very good actors . . . These were well-respected hospitals and doctors. And addicts are just really good liars. We're very good at getting what we want . . . it's more common than anybody knows.

In real life, that woman is a white, fifty-year-old mother of two college-aged sons who lives in a middle-class community. She is your average suburban neighbor. For emphasis, let me repeat: she says she got away with doctor shopping because she "didn't look like an addict." Doctors are just as prone to stereotyping as anyone else. In our collective minds, we've created the "image" of a drug addict and that image is usually a poor, inner-city black or Latino. Those are, for the most part, the people being imprisoned for drugs . . . illegal drugs. But if the statistics on overdoses are any indication, the reality is America's average drug addict today is increasingly a prescription-pill-popping middle-class Caucasian with a family and career.

La Vida Lohan

Troubled movie star Lindsay Lohan had already gone through three rehabs, two DUIs, reckless driving, and cocaine use when the courts finally seemed to be cracking down on her.[17] A judge ruled she'd violated probation by missing several court-ordered alcohol education classes and ordered her to jail, where she served thirteen days. But a probation officer's report revealed the real problem, noting Lindsay "takes the following prescription drugs: Nexium, Zoloft, trazadone (Desyrel), Adderall, and sometimes Dilaudid for dental pain."[18]

Hello?! Dilaudid has been compared in strength to morphine and heroin. Even as it seemed like the whole world was begging her to get clean, her probation officer's report concluded her testing "positive for amphetamines and opiates" was "not a violation of probation."[19] The lawyer for Lindsay's dad wrote an angry letter to California's attorney general complaining of "reports that she is able to call up doctors, and obtain whatever she wants, in whatever quantities she wants, whenever she wants. She can ingest these substances in jail . . . and on probation while subject to random drug tests, as prescription drugs are allowed. It's a giant loophole that could cost her her life."[20] That the courts thought these drugs were medically necessary and therefore okay reveals just how little our criminal justice system knows about drug abuse and how druggies cop their stash.

Sometimes the Drugs Are Just a Mouse Click Away

An addict with a laptop can find rogue Internet pharmacies that offer a simple online questionnaire in place of a visit to a flesh-and-blood doctor or let you talk to their doctor on the phone. In 2003, an FDA official told a congressional committee, "A patient-doctor relationship, in many cases, is never established. Attempts to stop some U.S. doctors and online pharmacies from issuing online prescriptions without a physical examination have not always been successful."[21] While there are many legitimate online pharmacies that do it right, the anonymity associated with the Internet could certainly feel like a protective cover for addicts who don't want someone in a white coat studying them when they request their refills.

"The fact that companies on the Internet can call my client—who is addicted—to try to seduce her to buy more pills is a crime, an absolute crime."

—Howard Samuels, Psy.D., licensed clinical psychologist, founder, and CEO of the Hills Treatment Center

After appearing on *Issues*, Nikki, the recovering prescription pill addict, talked me through the clever ways addicts use the World Wide Web to get high. "I went on this website. If you pay them one hundred seventy-five dollars, they send you a six-page list of pharmacies in Mexico and elsewhere. You call them and you speak to their pharmacist and they will send you a prescription from that country."

Those willing to physically trek into Mexico find it's a breeze to score. Mexican border towns are chock full of pharmacies that cater to American customers, often middle-class addicts hunting to get high. Nikki regaled me with stories of her drug-seeking forays south of the border. "I was in Mexico and I went to a pharmacy to get Valium, and Xanax sticks, and I was also able to get Percocet and Vicodin. But when I asked for OxyContin they sent me three blocks away to a hole-in-the-wall doctor's office up a flight of stairs. I gave the doctor fifty dollars and he gave me a prescription for 120 OxyContin, and then I went back to the pharmacy and paid cash for the pills."

Woodstock Redux

I'm not a Christian Scientist. I believe there's a good reason for doctors and legitimate medicine. I go to my doctors regularly and take prescriptions when I need them for absolute medical necessities. I am grateful for the level of health care that I'm lucky enough to receive. However, there's a growing trend in America to try to solve all manner of discomfort, real or imagined, physical or emotional, with a pill. That tendency has morphed into a cultural addiction.

"In the addict's mind it's okay because it was prescribed by a doctor, so it makes it easier to cross that line of addiction. In my private practice I've noticed that six or eight years ago the drug of choice was heroin and crystal meth where I would intervene. Today I would say it is 30 percent alcohol, 10 percent cocaine and crystal meth, and 60 percent prescription drugs."

–Ken Seeley, addiction expert and founder of Intervention 911

It's my belief that Big Pharma has long had a plan for us baby boomers who've come limping into the valley of middle age filled with vague aches and pains. The pharmaceutical industry is keenly aware that the Woodstock generation (and the disco generation after it) have always had a love affair with drugs. Big Pharma has simply figured out a way to make the drugs legal.

The legality of powerful, mind-altering medications gives boomers deniability. While they once smoked pot and dropped acid (or later did coke), today their long hair is shorn and gray and they've transformed themselves into "upstanding" citizens with "respectable" jobs and kids who need to be put through college. The hazy memories of wild nights partying are filed away in a little box in the closet to be forgotten. However, what has *not* gone away is the boomers' need to stuff their pain. Along with their respective individual traumas (divorce, job struggles, family conflicts, toxic secrets), the boomers, in particular, feel the need to self-medicate to fill the void in their lives. I happen to be one of those addicts, and that's why I'm in recovery.

Most of us boomers experienced a period of intense idealism in our youth where we really sought to understand the meaning of life and make our lives count, in a way that our parents had not. We wanted to be authentic! We wanted to change the world. We marched and chanted! We were the peaceniks who questioned authority and spoke truth to power. But as we took our place in the world and became the authority figures ourselves, the peace signs got tossed in the circular file and the bohemian minimalism of a spiritual life gave way to a craving for material comforts and status.

In other words, many—if not most—boomers sold out. Our rebel anthems have become the soundtracks for TV commercials. There is a subtle hollowness to the success many boomers have achieved, be they bankers, developers, lawyers, or some other species of professional. Some have made big money but, by caving in to an ego-based definition of success, have allowed their core values to become corrupted. As their stock portfolios fattened, many secretly careened into spiritual bankruptcy, which is a symptom of addiction. In fact, addiction to materialism dovetails neatly with addiction to prescription pills. It's a classic cross-addiction. The obsession with materialism leads to depression, which leads to antidepressants.

Peter Singer, professor of bioethics at Princeton University, has written a thought-provoking book called *The Life You Can Save*, arguing that Americans who would instinctively stop to save a drowning man are also morally obligated to help the millions dying of poverty around the world (whom they can't see) by tithing a significant percentage of their income to charity. "We might say that the rich have a right to spend their money on lavish parties, Patek Philippe watches, private jets, luxury yachts, and space travel, or, for that matter, to flush wads of it down the toilet. Or that those of us with more modest means shouldn't be forced to forgo any of the less expensive pleasures that offer us some relief from all the time we spend working. But we could still think that to choose to do these things rather than use the money to save human lives is wrong, shows a deplorable lack of empathy, and means that you are not a good person."[22]

That's a harsh assessment. But there's a sliver of unpleasant truth somewhere in there that we just don't want to face. How do we stuff these secret feelings of shame over the morally corrupt choices we've made? By self-medicating.

Where Have All the Hippies Gone? To the Pharmacy!

Instead of bellbottoms and beads, they're in khakis and reading glasses. Instead of grass and LSD, they've got medicine cabinets filled with Valium, Vicodin, Prozac, Effexor, Paxil, Zoloft, Percocet, Wellbutrin, Xanax, OxyContin, or Ambien . . . to name a few.

Playing Doctor

A sexy, soothing woman's voice explains how she's taking an antidepressant but thinks she still might need a little something extra to help with her moodiness. An authoritative announcer explains how most people who are being treated for depression still experience symptoms of depression. The voiceover artist explains that one antidepressant alone just might not be enough. The viewer is urged to consider asking his or her doctor to add on . . . (name that drug).

I am paraphrasing an actual commercial for an antidepressant currently on the market. Now this is a drug with a slew of potential side effects, from confusion to seizures to thoughts of suicide to uncontrollable muscle movements and even trouble swallowing.[23]

If you take just a moment to ponder these commercials, it should become obvious that the whole concept of direct advertising of prescription drugs to consumers is problematic! It's essentially asking people—who are not doctors themselves—to play doctor! "Ask your doctor about (insert drug)" is the suggestion at the heart of each and every one of these ads.

Some commercials don't even ask you to remember the name of their drug, saying, "Ask your doctor about the 'purple pill.'" That's easy enough, right? Here's the obvious problem with that: *Doctors* are supposed to diagnose your problem and offer what *they* think is the best medical treatment! They are not supposed to be in the business of entertaining uneducated suggestions from their patients. But doctors obviously do. Otherwise, the airwaves wouldn't be awash with these commercials and drug companies wouldn't be spending billions on these ads. This is self-medicating one step removed. Self-medication is the essence of addiction.

A Harvard/MIT study confirmed this, concluding that every dollar the pharmaceutical industry spent on direct-to-consumer advertising in the year 2000 yielded an additional $4.20 in drug sales.[24] Prescription drug use in America is skyrocketing! The amount Americans are spending on prescription pills has increased at a stunning rate over the last couple of decades, careening toward the $300 billion mark. But are we getting healthier and happier as a result? I think you could argue that the answer is no.

The biggest selling prescription drugs fight high cholesterol, which can also usually be lowered without drugs by simple dietary changes like reducing or eliminating meat and dairy products.[25] But it seems pharmaceutical companies would rather continue repackaging the same tired solutions in a capsule. A network news investigation concludes, "Much of the profits from prescription sales are not derived from breakthrough drugs, but rather from drugs that are similar to already popular medications."[26]

Depressed Celebrities

When you add a celebrity into the mix as the promoter of the drug, then you maximize the manipulation. This is exactly what's happening on TV and in print. A *New York Times* exposé noted that *Sopranos* shrink Lorraine Bracco talked about her depression and use of Zoloft while under a deal with Pfizer, the maker of Zoloft.[27] Former Pittsburgh Steelers quarterback Terry Bradshaw did a campaign dubbed "The Terry Bradshaw Depression Tour," sponsored by GlaxoSmithKline, which makes the antidepressants Wellbutrin and Paxil.[28] During that campaign, Bradshaw was quoted as saying, "The beauty of it is that there are medications that work. Look at me. I'm always happy-go-lucky, and people look at me and find it shocking that I could be depressed."[29]

The star-studded list of prescription pitch artists goes on and on. The *New York Times* notes, "Most of the celebrity antidepressant promotions are unbranded, meaning the television commercials do not mention the product by name, but often refer consumers to a website that does."[30] The bottom line? They are singing a siren song to lead customers down a pathway to the drug. We all know consumers are more likely to buy a product if they think a star is using it too. As a branding strategist told the *New York Times*, "The reality is people want a piece of something they can't be . . . They live vicariously through the products and services that those celebrities are tied to. Years from now, our descendants may look at us and say, 'God, these were the most gullible people who ever lived.'"[31]

There is a growing consensus that it's insidious to use celebrities to hock antidepressants, which can have serious side effects and are prone to abuse, to the general public. Critics say the worst part is that it's sometimes not clear if and when stars are being paid by a drug company to share their health story with the public. When

Kathleen Turner appeared on national television to talk about her battle with rheumatoid arthritis, many viewers probably did not realize she was reportedly being paid by drug companies that sell a drug to treat rheumatoid arthritis.[32] Now, many networks are going out of their way to ask stars, beforehand, if they're pitching for a drug company and will tell viewers about any ties they uncover. If only Uncle Sam were as vigilant.

The Food and Drug Administration is supposed to regulate drug companies but often behaves more like a shill for the drug industry, looking out for the industry's interests even when they conflict with the interests of consumers. In 2000, a *USA Today* exposé found "more than half of the experts hired to advise the government on the safety and effectiveness of medicine have financial relationships with the pharmaceutical companies that will be helped or hurt by their decisions . . . The conflicts typically include stock ownership, consulting fees or research grants." Following a barrage of criticism, the FDA has tightened its rules to bar anyone with a conflicting financial interest of over fifty thousand dollars from serving on its advisory committees, but there continues to be a complex waiver system that is ripe for manipulation.[33]

The United States government needs to get out of bed with Big Pharma and end the incestuous relationship between the FDA and drug makers. But that's not likely to happen as long as the drug industry retains its chokehold on Washington. The Pharmaceutical Researchers and Manufacturers of America (PhRMA) is the largest single-industry lobbying group in America. Big Pharma has more lobbyists than there are members of both houses of Congress![34] So, until lobbyists are banned, which isn't likely to happen any time soon, it's up to the consumer to make less self-destructive choices.

Sitting Through the Feelings

The proliferation of antidepressants, antianxiety drugs, and painkillers raises a profound philosophical question. Should we try to avoid pain or . . . just experience it? Let's remove from the discourse the obvious extremes. If a person is suffering excruciating pain from a burn injury or major surgery, they obviously need to take advantage of something that will prevent their moment-to-moment existence from becoming intolerable torture. Ditto for psychological crisis. If someone is suicidal and there's a drug to keep them from killing themselves, then it clearly makes sense.

What I'm questioning are the less extreme physical and psychological ailments. If someone is suffering the kind of depression that is not severe enough to keep them from eating, sleeping, and working, should they try to blot out the sadness they are experiencing . . . or should they try to figure out why they're sad and try to fix what's wrong? The biggest problem with antidepressants and antianxiety pills is that they don't fix the underlying problem that's making you depressed and anxious! So when you try to get off the pills, the sadness and anxiety return. Then you go back on the pills and . . . become hooked!

What we call depression is often nature's warning bell that something is out of balance and needs to be corrected. Often that "problem" is not something we can see, hear, smell, touch, or taste. It's often an emotional or psychological problem: an unresolved childhood trauma, a skewed view of how the world operates, a simmering resentment, a toxic relationship, or a distorted perception of self. A woman who is "blue" and is told to take antidepressants may actually be trapped in a loveless marriage that she should end. If she takes medication to numb herself, then she is simply prolonging her problem and postponing judgment day for her relationship. She is certainly not confronting the real crisis in her life. A young man who is depressed may actually be deeply unfulfilled by the soulless career that he has chosen. Taking medication allows him to remain glued to a computer while trapped inside a cubicle all day. However, he's betraying himself by taking a drug that makes that bad choice tolerable.

Children Should Be Seen and Not Heard?

I'm absolutely convinced that if I were a kid today, I would be diagnosed with attention deficit/hyperactivity disorder (ADHD), and a doctor would be pushing my parents to get me on meds to calm me down. As a kid, I was beyond hyperactive and extremely mischievous. Basically, I was acting out a lot. Some of that had to do with growing up in an alcoholic household. Like most kids who get into trouble, I was unconsciously expressing anger that had no other outlet. It's a common story. So is the best solution to sedate the child . . . or to confront the dysfunction in the home? Obviously, it's a lot easier to numb the child than to deal with the messy family issues underneath the misbehavior.

While rich and even middle-class kids often have the luxury of psychological therapy, where they can talk out their problems, poor children do not. Studies show children covered by Medicaid are given powerful antipsychotic meds at a rate four times higher than kids whose parents have private insurance. These Medicaid kids are more likely to get drugs for less severe conditions than middle-class kids. These drugs have serious side effects, often causing drastic weight gain and producing lifelong physical problems. Antipsychotic drugs are now being used on about 300,000 minors in America. It's such a problem that a group of Medicaid professionals has formed a group called Too Many, Too Much, Too Young.[35]

Kids First, Then You and Me

Given the trend of ever-increasing drug use, is it really all that far-fetched to imagine a gray future where everybody is on mood-altering substances for one reason or another? In this heavily sedated future, medication might even be "required" not just for unruly children but also for rebellious segments of the adult population. The opiate of the masses may well turn out to be prescribed! As it stands now, a stunning one out of every two Americans is on some sort of prescription medication.[36] How long before it's two out of two?

Pharming

So how do we reverse this insidious trend? First, let's avoid becoming our children's primary drug supplier. Within the prescription drug abuse crisis, there's another epidemic of teenagers stealing their parents mood-altering meds. Today, more teens are beginning their drug experimentation by abusing prescription pills than by smoking pot. Federal drug officials say three-quarters of teenagers get pills from a friend or relative. Less than 5 percent get prescription pills from a drug dealer or other stranger.[37] The five prescription drugs kids most frequently steal from their parents' medicine cabinet are: painkillers like OxyContin, stimulants like Ritalin, sedatives like Valium, sleep aids like Ambien, and cough medicines.[38] The latest teen fad? "Cabinet parties." A police chief in California described it this way, "Teens raid their parents' medicine cabinet for opiates such as Vicodin and OxyContin, and take them to the party, where the pills are dumped into a large bowl for communal use."[39] Kids haphazardly dip into the pills in the bowl, which they call "trail mix." The whole process is called "pharming." Very funny . . . until it kills someone. Experts suggest we get rid of any old prescription bottles. Parents are also urged to literally lock up their medicine cabinet the way they would a rifle. Both can be deadly.

But perhaps the best way to discourage your kids from popping pills is to not pop them yourself. If teenagers see their parents medicating themselves through a career or family mess, that's what they're likely to do when confronted with a problem.

We Must Learn to Embrace Our Suffering and Let It Teach Us Something

Sometimes I think depression is a natural state. We'd like to be perpetually happy. But suffering is an intrinsic part of the human experience. Most often I find when I'm feeling depressed, it's because I'm self-obsessed. Egocentricity is inherently alienating because it's a "me"—separate from everyone else—attitude. Recovery programs teach the addict to "get out of your own head" and help someone else. When I forget about myself, I realize I'm a small part of a larger entity called the universe and therefore my alienation turns to empathy for those with whom I share the universe. They say all we can get is a daily reprieve from addiction. Perhaps all we can get is a daily respite from the depression inherent in us, not by taking drugs, but by recognizing that we are part of a larger whole and acting in a way that benefits everyone, not just ourselves.

It would also help if we got out of our denial over the extent of prescription drug abuse in America. When *Clueless* actress Brittany Murphy died, many in Hollywood immediately assumed it was drug related. Her mother was furious, telling *People* magazine her daughter was merely "high on life."[40] The coroner ultimately concluded her death was accidental due to pneumonia and iron deficiency

anemia but with multiple-drug intoxication—all prescription drugs—
as a contributing factor.[41]

Obviously, I have compassion for a grieving mother. But this
would appear to be classic codependency. We must deal with the big
elephant in the room and confront any loved one who is using even
a single prescription pill for an invalid reason. Tough love is never
fun. But consider the alternative.

Chapter Three
THE CYBERS: Addicted to Tech

It's hot in Reno, Nevada. But a man and a woman in their early twenties are blind to the weather outside. They are not even conscious of being on this planet. Michael and Iana Straw are living in a parallel universe. Their portal to this other world? The Internet. And where, in this fantasy landscape, have they staked their claim? In the cyberland known as Dungeons & Dragons, which has been described as the "most realistic combat system of any online game," where you play with your "unique and highly customizable" D&D character, fighting "bad-ass monsters and dragons" and evading "traps left by an ancient race," all in "vast and dangerous" Eberron.[1]

Back on planet Earth, off in the corner of the Straw's home, their two little children slowly starve. Cops say the Straw's toddler son and infant daughter were severely malnourished and near death when social workers rushed them to a hospital. "They had food; they just chose not to give it to their kids because they were too busy playing video games," the prosecutor said of the parents, who pleaded guilty to child neglect. Their two children were put in foster care.[2]

We all know how drugs and alcohol can lead to child abuse. But how can anyone be so completely hooked on a *game* that they let their kids starve in RL (*real life* in cyberspeak)?

Like most drugs, online gaming presents itself as the solution, when it's really the problem. In *Unplugged: My Journey Into the Dark*

World of Video Game Addiction, Ryan Van Cleave explains that, as an addicted player's real life deteriorates "the playing of online games can (somewhat paradoxically) help the player numb, destress, relax, and 'zone out.'"[3] The author is a recovering gaming addict himself, who once contemplated suicide over it, and explains why it can become impossible to walk away from the game. It comes from the expectation and anticipation of the next reward or point, which the player always hopes is just a click or two away. These games are brilliantly designed with the promise of another point always on the horizon. *Oh, just a few more minutes in Eberron and then I'll feed the kids.*

A Complicated Cultural Contagion

Cyberaddiction is perhaps the most complex societal contagion America is facing today because the nature of the Internet is so complex and all encompassing. Along with online gaming, there is e-mail, texting, Twitter, Facebook, MySpace, YouTube, Skype, Google, Yahoo, LinkedIn, iTunes, eBay, Amazon, Craigslist, Tumblr, innumerable chat rooms, and something like 240 million other websites, a number that just keeps skyrocketing.[4] The portal to cyberspace can be a desktop, a laptop, a BlackBerry, an iPhone, various other smartphones, an iPad, or a Kindle. "Internet clouds" now exist where a person's files can be stored in cyberspace to be viewed from any Internet-accessible device anywhere in the world. Hasta la vista, clogged hard drive. Never again will we be tethered to only one computer.

"When I'm playing a game, everything stops and I have something to focus on. It's like a meditation. I get relief from thoughts of the oil spill, my budget and income, my age, the end of the world, my mother, where I would rather live, why I can't buy property, and how will I retire. Playing a game over and over gives me a sense of control in a world that feels entirely out of my control."

—April East, online gaming addict

The Internet Is Truly Becoming a Whole New World

When it comes to escaping, nothing beats an alternate world, especially one where you can assume any identity you want and create an alter ego. Many games encourage you to reinvent yourself in the form of an avatar that you can imbue with all sorts of powerful, daring, and desirable physical characteristics that—in real life—you may not have. Could you slay a towering dragon if it appeared before you in real life?

The Internet Is a Portal to All Manner of Addictive Behavior

They talk about pot being a gateway drug to hard drugs, which I don't necessarily believe. But I do believe that the Internet can be an easy-access entryway to gambling addiction, sex addiction, workaholism, prescription drug abuse, compulsive texting, and celebrity obsession. Every aspect of our lives that the Internet touches, it transforms. Bye-bye CDs, DVDs, newspapers, magazines, books, dictionaries, encyclopedias, maps, bank tellers, etc., etc., etc. In the same manner, the World Wide Web has transformed our cravings, making it easier than ever before to get more of what we're jonesing for.

"We all know that screen media is habituating. It's hard to pull ourselves away from our computers. Screen media is incredibly compelling."

—Susan Linn, Ed.D., director of the Campaign for a Commercial-Free Childhood

The Internet Has Supersized
and Accelerated Our Addictions

Take gambling. In just the last decade, online poker websites have gone from making virtually no money to raking in about $5 billion a year. The new cyber-trained poker players study their laptops. The hand they are dealt is not nearly as important as the stats they are processing at lightning speed. And that's precisely why they are quickly turning the old-fashioned, instinctive poker players—who trust their gut—into a joke. It's no longer about bluffing and reading the telltale expressions of your opponents. Today, a good poker face is a pasty mug that has spent many hours staring at a computer screen mastering probability and patterns. While the old-style poker champs would play in a couple of dozen tournaments a year, the new cyber-poker players can knock that out online in one night, accumulating heaps of information upon which to base their betting decisions. This revolution in poker was laid out in a fascinating *Time* magazine article, "World Series of Poker: Attack of the Math Brats," which profiled a "new breed of math nerd, those guys using a mountain of sortable data from the millions of hands played online to dominate the game."[5] These new hot shots are not pretending to be emotionless. They are emotionless. They basically have little regard for how bad a hand they have because, says *Time*, they "rely on online software, which tracks every move and provides instant feedback on how a player is likely to respond." For them, it's truly a numbers game.

But for every mathematically gifted professional gambler who treats it as a job, there are thousands of amateur gamblers out there who are losing their paychecks, their homes, their relationships, and their self-respect to a gambling addiction that no longer requires a drive to a casino or a smoke-filled backroom. The temptation is now a mere click of the mouse away.

Leaving Las Vegas

Even the most inveterate traditional poker player eventually has to fold 'em so he can sleep, eat, change his clothes, or go to the bathroom. But the Internet player can literally take his gambling table into the kitchen, the bedroom, or the bathroom. Imagine a full-blown alcoholic locked inside a liquor store. That's what it's like for a gambling addict at home or the office. The casino is living with him, as an ever-present virtual reality.

Gambling is skyrocketing in the United States. It's particularly on the rise among young people. The Internet is a huge reason. It may not feel quite as sleazy to lose a game on your home computer as it does to lose at a table filled with badly dressed people in a raggedy casino on the edge of the Las Vegas strip. But money lost is money lost. The average debt of a male pathological gambler in America is between fifty-five and ninety grand. The stress and anxiety of this addiction can be fatal. Experts say one in five pathological gamblers attempts suicide.[6]

The Internet Magnifies the Addictive
Nature of a Substance or Behavior

In recovery we are told to stay away from people, places, and things that can trigger an addictive craving. Recovering alcoholics often avoid the bars where they used to get drunk. Recovering drug addicts often sidestep the corner stoop where they know their old pusher is hanging out, ever ready to lure them back into their disease. But there's no running away from the Internet. Most of us are required to use the Internet at work, and increasingly, it's becoming an indispensible part of our home life. We hop on to find a takeout restaurant, e-mail a friend, or advertise on Craigslist.

Practical and harmless, right? Not if you're a sex addict.

The Internet Turbocharges Sex Addiction

If you're a sex addict, the Internet is like having a mistress, a brothel, a dungeon, an orgy, a sex slave, a dominatrix, and every manner of fetish device ever invented at the tip of your fingers 24/7/365. Now that's temptation. *Cybersex addiction* is a subcategory of both sex addiction and Internet addiction. I would call cybersex addiction a blended cross-addiction, where two addictions merge into one compulsive behavior. Estimates are one in five Internet addicts are engaged in some kind of online sexual behavior, either watching porn, having cybersex, or seducing someone in a chat room.[7]

There are currently an estimated 5 to 6 million adult websites.[8] It took me less than a minute on my laptop to get to serious hard-core, triple X–rated porn. I simply Googled "top adult websites," clicked on Adultreviews.com, and was presented with links to various featured sites like PornstarsPunishment.com (which is exactly what the title suggests it will be). Clicking on another link, Penisbot.com, brought me to dozens of categories of graphic porn. The site features dozens of different fetishes, all possible orientations, uniforms, combinations, positions, and activities including BDSM, which stands for *bondage/discipline/sadomasochism,* along with practices simply too extreme to mention in this book. In a matter of a few minutes I saw dozens of extraordinarily graphic still photos, video trailers, and short films often culminating with what they call "the money shot."

The proliferation of webcams have also brought us what are called "chat models" or "cam girls," who perform erotic acts, often naked, in real time before a webcam on a pay-per-view basis. A whole industry—complete with videochat studios—has cropped up around these "private shows."[9]

Sex is one of the most pleasurable and electrifying aspects of the human experience and, hence, can easily become very addictive, even when done the old-fashioned way . . . in person. I don't consider myself a sex addict. Still, I have to be honest. I had a hard time pulling myself away from some of the triple-X imagery that is simultaneously revolting and mesmerizing. Knowing what I know about addiction, if sex were my drug of choice I think I would be surfing porn for hours or even days on end. The Internet offers the kind of extreme sexual acts it would be hard to arrange in real life.

The Online Sex Addict Rapidly Develops a Tolerance for Porn

When an addict develops a tolerance for the standard fare, that means he or she will require ever more graphic imagery to achieve the same state of arousal. This is where the Internet experience differs from the real-world experience. In the real world, things end, whether it's a live porn show, a lap dance, or an hour with a hooker. In the virtual world, there is no end! There is always another website with another porn video or another webcam show at the next click. And there's complete access to that next addictive rush.

All addicts build up a tolerance for their drug of choice. The more they have of it, the more of it they need to experience an equivalent high. This progressive vicious cycle is accelerated on the Internet. Just as the online gambler plays in one night what the quaint old-world gambler plays in a year, so an online sex addict can build up a tolerance on the Web that would take him years if he stuck to real contact with real flesh-and-blood sex partners. So a porn addict is liable to need ever greater amounts of ever more stimulating porn, which is liable to take that person into some extremely disturbing content. All addiction leads to moral bankruptcy, and online sex addiction is one of the more florid examples of that principle.

The Internet Creates Faux Intimacy

Next to porn, one of the largest categories of paid content on the Web is online dating.[10] Addiction to cyberdating is a growing phenomenon, and women are particularly susceptible. Match.com, JDate.com, Chemistry.com . . . these are just some of the dating sites that have become household names. But some of the lesser known sites offer more insight into the deeper motivations behind many online daters' machinations.

One particularly candid dating site begins by reminding the visitor of the old saying that it's just as easy to fall in love with a rich man as a poor one. It tells the prospective female "Sugar Baby" that she deserves to be treated like a princess and to have successful men make her life easier and better financially. And it promises that all this can be arranged within a few minutes. There is a picture of a beautiful female described as ambitious, affectionate, and in need of pampering by a classy, mature man. A photo of a handsome older man projects affluence and generosity. He offers to mentor, pamper, and spoil the right woman. I'll let you do the math on that equation. The site claims to have 2 million members and says it's inundated with men and women trying to join.

Millions of Americans now come home from work only to dive into their laptops, eager to see what responses have come in from their dating profile listings and to flirt via online chat with their new prospects. But all too often, the hours spent engaged in sexual intrigue are wasted by the lies and distortions of two strangers, who've never met, trying to impress each other with the best photo they've ever taken while robbed of their most effective communications skills. We've all heard the expression, 99 percent of communication is nonverbal. When we chat online, we vainly attempt to get a read on someone without the benefit of any of our natural instincts and intuitive tools, namely sight, sound, smell, and touch. The cyber chatterbox who brags of slaying dragons in a chat room might well be terrified of a firefly in RL, but how would we know that from the tap, tap, tap of his fingertips?

No Face Time

There's a very dangerous trend that's an outgrowth of cyber addiction. There is growing resistance, among all of us, to engage in face-to-face communication. American teens now use their cell phones, computers, video games, and TV for almost eight hours a day. Add in multitasking and the figure is even higher.[11] So kids are spending the equivalent of an adult's entire workday with their nose in some sort of electronic media, tuning out the natural world around them.

> "I was driving with my daughter down this country road. And while driving, there was this beautiful scenery outside, but she's in the car staring at this little screen on her cell phone. There is a risk of losing a connection with the natural world in favor of a connection with a piece of technology."
>
> —*Anonymous mom*

In some circles, talking is actually becoming uncool. Today's young teens consider gabbing on the phone old hat and have replaced a lot of in-person and voice communication with texting. Half of American teens send fifty or more text messages a day. One-third of them send more than 100 texts per day.[12] Think about it: 100 texts a day from a kid who is still in school? That's laying the foundation for addictive behavior. I've covered news stories where parents have been assaulted by their own children when they tried to take away the kid's cell phone. That sounds a lot like the fierce defiance of an addict who will fight to keep his or her drug of choice, no matter what.

Facebook and other social-networking sites have taken the place of in-your-face conversation. Twitter, the act of posting short personal texts to a group of followers, may seem like a ridiculous idea at first glance. After all, who really wants to hear that someone just picked up their dry cleaning or is late to the dentist? But millions of Americans have fallen in love with the notion of sharing their every thought in 140 characters or less. This has spawned an entirely new way of communicating. Kids, especially, have learned to replace the nuances of in-person communication with symbols, flash icons, and even keyboard art. Acronyms, shorthand spelling, slang, and capitalization are writing styles that have taken the place of body language, expressions, and voice. These short bursts of communication are known as microblogging. Social scientists call the ability to feel close to others via cyberspace communication alone "ambient awareness."[13]

"This is the paradox of ambient awareness. Each little update—each individual bit of social information—is insignificant on its own, even supremely mundane. But taken together, over time, the little snippets coalesce into a surprisingly sophisticated portrait of your friends' and family members' lives, like thousands of dots making a pointillist painting."

—*Clive Thompson, columnist for* Wired

But is communicating primarily through computers dangerous to our mental health? A *New York Times* article aptly titled "Antisocial

Networking?" suggests "today's youths may be missing out on experiences that help them develop empathy, understand emotional nuances and read social cues like facial expressions and body language."[14] On my show, *Issues*, we covered a horrific story that proves there's good reason to be worried that obsessive texting can lead to callousness and cruelty.

March 17, 2010. It's another gorgeous day in Deerfield Beach, Florida. Fifteen-year-old Josie Ratley has just left her classes for the afternoon. She is at the school's bus loop waiting to go home. Out of nowhere, a fifteen-year-old boy named Wayne Treacy storms up to her. He appears enraged. Cops say he begins to viciously beat the girl, pummeling her until she falls to the ground, then smashing her head onto the pavement, kicking her, and stomping on her face with his steel-toed boots, leaving her near death.

Doctors say every single bone in Josie's face was broken in that attack. When she emerged from three weeks in a medically induced coma she was unable to speak or walk. She also suffered extensive and traumatic brain injury that required three surgeries on her skull. She will need long-term rehabilitative care.

Her Life Was Destroyed . . . All Over a Text Message

Prosecutors say Wayne Treacy had become incensed over a text message that Josie Ratley had sent Wayne referring to his brother, who had recently committed suicide. Hours before the beating, cops say Wayne began texting his friends about how he planned to retaliate against the girl for her text. Court documents paint a portrait of a young man whose texts are overflowing with rage. "Snap her neck then stomp her skull. Fastest way I could think of," he allegedly wrote, describing his plan of attack. In another text sent about an hour before the beating, he purportedly writes, "This bxtch ran her mouth bout my bro who she knew is dead. Nao I want her head." Prosecutors say Wayne's final text was "I just tried to kill sum1. Im going to prison." He was charged as an adult with first-degree attempted murder.[15]

If this young man had done less texting and engaged in more genuine conversation or, better yet, shared his pain over his brother's suicide with a trained therapist, would his rage have built up to this level? As obsessive texting becomes a substitution for talking, we are likely to see more explosions of sudden violence from people who are not giving themselves an outlet to express and process their feelings.

> "Our bodies are built for 'fight or flight.' We are supposed to go out and do things physically every day but don't. We just sit there vibrating. Then we get these adrenaline surges but have nowhere to let it out. It drives us crazy. We have not adapted physically to our new virtual world."
>
> —*April East, Internet gaming addict*

Cyber Sadism

There is a sense that cyberspace is a no-consequence zone. Not true. The anonymity of the Internet gives many people a perverse courage to be their worst selves. Teens routinely text, e-mail, and post nasty things about each other that they would never have the courage to say to someone's face. One girl told the *New York Times*, "It's easier to fight online, because you feel more brave and in control . . . on Facebook, you can be as mean as you want."[16] Of course, she's right. It's a lot easier to write "you're such a slut" than to say those same words to someone's face. The Cyberbullying Research Center says it found that one in five middle-school students are being bullied via the Internet or text. One in five! That's a cyberbullying epidemic![17] Vicious sexual comments, ethnic and racial slurs, and derogatory references to income and class are common. Often kids can do it anonymously.

To stay one step ahead of their parents, kids often jump from one social-networking site to another. Formspring.me is a relatively new social-networking site that was singled out by the *New York Times* as "a magnet for comments, many of them nasty and sexual, among the Facebook generation . . . it has become an obsession for thousands of teenagers nationwide, a place to trade comments and questions like: Are you still friends with julia? Why wasn't sam invited to lauren's party? You're not as hot as u think u are. Do you wear a d cup? You talk too much. You look stupid when you laugh."[18]

When a seventeen-year-old Long Island girl committed suicide in March 2010, cops wondered if the vicious taunts she had received on social-networking sites might have been a factor. Perhaps most horrifying, the online taunts continued even after her death. "She was obviously a stupid depressed—who deserved to kill herself. she got what she wanted. be happy for her death. rejoice in it," someone wrote.[19] One parent whose child was a friend of the victim noted, "There are posts of photos with nooses around her neck. It's disgusting and heartless."

Does this callousness have an addictive component? Of course! We know that teens are texting 50 to 100 times a day and then posting a slew of other messages on social-networking sites. That's called being hooked. We know that addiction leads to moral bankruptcy. Alcoholism, for example, routinely leads to domestic violence in the home with spouses, kids, and even pets brutalized by the drunk family patriarch. Kids are not immune to this phenomenon of addiction-based cruelty. Addiction creates a single-mindedness that kills every other voice inside one's head, silencing the conscience.

There is a growing obsession with being the cool, cold texter with the pithy putdown. Since all addictive behavior is progressive, it follows that the anonymous comments will become nastier as the teen's texting addiction spirals out of control. This is a social contagion of the first order! So where are the adults? Getting and sending e-mails on their CrackBerrys, of course. Remember the first time you heard "You've got mail!"?

Ping! Ping! Ping!

It's the tantalizing sound that tells us somebody is knocking on our cyberdoor. There's that moment of suspense as we wonder . . . *Is it her? Is it him? Is it that good news I've been waiting for? Is it that bad news I've been fearing? Who is it? What do they want?* That moment of anticipation as we scramble to open the message gives us a dopamine rush. Dopamine, a chemical similar to adrenaline, influences our ability to experience pleasure or pain. It's the same kind of rush a gambler gets as the roulette wheel spins. *Where will it land? What will I win? What might I lose?* And then, if the message is a winner, we get another hit of pleasure, another surge of dopamine. This is really what it's all about. Getting the rush from the ping!

I should know. I hear a lot of pings. Like many people who work in the news media, I have two BlackBerrys, one for work and one for personal use. I, too, text and e-mail dozens and dozens of times over the course of an average day. So am I a total hypocrite for beating my chest about cyberaddiction? Yes . . . and no. It always comes back to this: *What is my intention in using a given device to send a message?*

Let's All Get Honest About Why We're Hitting SEND

Two guys are standing on a street corner and each is holding a BlackBerry. Each is looking down and hitting SEND on an e-mail. They're both doing the exact same thing. However, one of them is engaging in addictive behavior and the other is not. The difference is the emotionally sober person has a healthy motive for his actions, while the addict is using the device as a form of escape. Here are some very common, unhealthy reasons people will whip out their BlackBerry or other smartphone and start fiddling:

- out of self-importance
- to flash a status symbol
- to escape boredom, depression, or other unpleasant feelings
- to send a passive-aggressive signal that you're not interested in what's going on around you or the people you're with
- to get a hit or buzz from the suspense of opening up an e-mail or text that's just come in
- to be a people pleaser as you worry that you've got to respond instantly or others won't like you
- to procrastinate, pushing off a more important task or project
- to fill time
- to appear busy
- to avoid self-reflection
- to avoid being present in the moment
- out of fear of intimacy
- to feel connected, thereby quashing feelings of alienation
- to combat loneliness
- to avoid looking like you are alone
- to imply that you are popular

I once did a pitch for a TV show to an arrogant, young network executive who looked down at his BlackBerry and scrolled through his e-mails the entire time I was talking. I wanted to jump over the table and smack him. He was clearly signaling to me that he had little to no interest in what I had to say and that I was wasting his time. I would have preferred him to say that flat out. Or . . . perhaps he was just a desperate CrackBerry addict hitting bottom.

CrackBerry Inventory

If you're worried that your texting, e-mailing, or posting has become out of control, a twelve-step inventory is always a great way to get some perspective on your behavior. Try counting how many times you check your e-mail and text messages and Facebook on a given day. (Hey, they should have an "app" for that!) Then ask yourself what percentage of those spot checks were really necessary? If you're neurotically checking work e-mails after hours, on weekends, and during vacations, you may be cross-addicted, hooked on the Internet and work. That's cyberworkaholism. If so, you're not alone. Most smartphone owners will admit to checking their business e-mails on weekends and on vacation. In fact, many of us become panicked if we accidentally leave our cell phones at home, making it impossible to relax.

Cyberworkaholism is a tricky blended addiction because it's often rewarded with career success, raises, promotions, and other perks, so on the surface, it doesn't seem like a problem. But, like all addiction, it will ultimately turn self-destructive. Handheld devices were supposed to untether us from our desks and give us the freedom to roam. But when the usage becomes compulsive, it can feel like you are dragging your entire office with you wherever you go.

Given that a BlackBerry can store 28,000 pages of information,[20] that's not such a wild exaggeration. Surveys have shown widespread resentment by spouses of smartphone owners who complain that they, and their children, are often competing with the device for the user's attention.

In a world where we realistically cannot throw our smartphones out the window, it really becomes about managing the gray areas by setting boundaries. For example, on weekends, I try to rely on my personal BlackBerry, figuring if there's a crisis at work, they'd know to call me on my personal phone. I also have learned to put my BlackBerrys on silent when I go into a twelve-step meeting or a solemn situation such as a funeral. Frankly, I learned that the hard way. It seems nobody wants to hear my "I Kissed a Girl" ringtone erupt as they're reciting the eulogy.

Multitasking . . . Really?

Here's the really big question. Is all this instant communication really making us more productive, or could it simply be overwhelming us with a tsunami of data? The company-supplied smartphone is said to give employers a massive return on their investment in the devices. Suddenly, they have workers who are making the most of previously dead time, furiously e-mailing in the elevator, while they're walking the halls, and even in the bathroom.

Most of us, in this Information Age, engage in some form of digital juggling. When I'm at work, I'm constantly jumping between two TV sets on two different news networks, two BlackBerrys with different e-mail lists, and a computer desktop with all sorts of other data, like news scripts and wire copy, not to mention that quaint, bulky phone with the old-school receiver on my desk.

What can I say? Screen media is seductive. They made it that way!

There are times when I can feel overwhelmed and even a tad disoriented. Call it the "where was I?" syndrome. When I stop one task, my mind has to exit from that subject and approach the other task. Then, when I return to the initial subject, I have to reorient my mind and figure out where I left off. All of that takes time and energy. Constantly dipping in and out of different subjects and hopping from one communication device to another can be a time waster that can create a synthetic form of attention deficit disorder. There is growing evidence now that more and more people are superficially skimming reading material as opposed to really studying a piece of writing from beginning to end.

Is the Breadth of Our Knowledge Expanding at the Expense of Its Depth?

The progressive nature of addiction is accelerating all these trends. It often seems that we have all been duped into becoming slaves to shiny gadgets just to make very rich people even richer. Our world is becoming smaller as we increasingly focus on the intricate, little gizmo in our hands, ignoring the big, exciting world around us. Meantime, the more information about ourselves we surrender, the more ammunition we give cyberpushers to control and manipulate us.

In the *Atlantic*, Nicholas Carr has a fascinating article entitled "Is Google Making Us Stupid?" He writes, "The faster we surf across the Web—the more links we click and pages we view—the more opportunities Google and other companies gain to collect information about us and to feed us advertisements. Most of the proprietors of the commercial Internet have a financial stake in collecting the crumbs of data we leave behind as we flit from link to link—the more crumbs, the better. The last thing these companies want is to encourage leisurely reading or slow, concentrated thought. It's in their economic interest to drive us to distraction."

It's ironic that the baby boomer generation would have heralded the age of digital multitasking and websurfing. It's the antithesis of the credo of our youth. In *Doing Nothing—A History of Loafers, Loungers, Slackers, and Bums in America,* Tom Lutz waxes poetic about the doing-nothing ethic of the 1960s cultural revolution.[21] He reminds us that we celebrated writers like Baba Ram Dass who told us that "striving, pushing, desperate grabbing at the brass ring—any and all ambitious desires—were worse than distractions; they were the very stuff that made nirvana impossible and were destroying the planet. One had to let go, drop out, be free." Baba Ram Dass sums it all up with this: "Now is now. Are you going to be here or not?"[22] That's the very question we need to ask ourselves the next time we hear our cell phone ping!

Chapter Four
THE STARGAZERS: Addicted to Celebrity

I am standing inside Madison Square Garden, one of the high citadels of celebrity worship. This is where pop superstars come to receive the genuflecting adoration of their swooning fans. I am here to bear witness to the newest goddess of the cybergeneration. Emerging from the darkness in a cloud of white smoke, Lady Gaga easily takes possession of the tens of thousands of us packed together in front of the stage. She orders us to drop the glowing cell phones we're all pointing at her to take pictures. Instead, she demands we wave our arms and scream out our love for her. "You should cheer from start to finish," she shouts! We obey giddily. We have surrendered to her and become her "little monsters." In between her explosively choreographed renditions of "Poker Face," "Bad Romance," and "Just Dance," Madonna's heir apparent switches from one extraordinarily ornate outfit to another. My favorite was a glittery one-piece swimsuit that shot long flames out of her breasts and crotch.

Lady Gaga also sprinkles in little speeches. "Tonight is proof to all of you that you can be whoever you want to be! [cheers] Because I used to be standing right there, where you are, looking up at some BITCH on the stage that I wanted to be!" To that, the sold-out crowd erupts as one in a monstrous roar, affirming her theatrically expressed thesis.

No wonder her album/tour is entitled *The Fame Monster* and one of her hits is "Paparazzi." Lady Gaga gets fame! She has just neatly summed up one key motive behind our collective addiction to celebrity.

We All Want to Be Stars

As if to confirm that Gaga has correctly psychoanalyzed the crowd, everywhere I look the stands are filled with mini-Gagas, young women—and some young men—wearing strange things on their heads and painting their faces with extreme makeup, trying hard to look and act as avant-garde as their idol.

Lady Gaga is up on that stage precisely because she thought up all that wild stuff—the outrageously deformed musical instruments, the fire-shooting outfits, the concept of clothing as movable sculpture, the playing of the piano with her feet and even her behind. Not to mention that it's hard to get her *rah, rah, ump pa pa* dance tunes out of your head. She may have borrowed some inspiration from other stars, including Madonna, Elton John, and David Bowie. But Lady Gaga is clearly an original.

> "The ingredients (for fame) are the indescribable and the special. People love authenticity and people love something that feels fresh."
>
> *—Perez Hilton, celebrity blogger*

When We See the Real Deal, We Know It

Originality is what makes a genuine star: inventing something new, combined with uncommon talent and having the guts to lay it all out there and act like you don't care if the world agrees. And sometimes the world doesn't agree. Not long after I attended her concert, I was one of many revolted by the now-infamous dress Lady Gaga wore to an awards show that was made of raw meat from a slaughtered animal. Determined to perpetually trump herself, she crossed the line into obscene cruelty. But the really scary part is that someone with Lady Gaga's enormous influence can inspire callousness in her fans, who want to be just like her. Many girls imitated her meat dress on Halloween.[1]

We Live Through Our Shining Star

The celebrity with whom we identify becomes our avatar in the rarified world occupied by the famous, allowing us to vicariously navigate it. We want to be that living, breathing model of success and drink in the adulation. Our imaginations exploit it to the max. In our subconscious there's a moment where we merge. That experience of feeling like the star ourselves causes a pleasure rush. Suddenly, the wiring gets crossed and—for a moment—we're supercharged. *We* are on stage, *we're* getting the wild applause, *we're* swamped by the paparazzi, and *we* are hustled along the red carpet past the nameless, faceless people whose pathetic club we desperately seek to escape. That's the addictive hit!

Admiring a genuine star like Lady Gaga, who comes along once in a blue moon, is one thing. But America is in the throes of a populist plague that has manifested itself in a feverish obsession with "celebrities" of all sizes, shades, and stripes, regardless of talent or originality. The explosion of media outlets—hundreds of cable channels, millions of websites—has created a plethora of platforms that people mount in order to declare their celebrity status. And the public co-signs it.

"The concept of being a celebrity has been cheapened. There are many more paths to celebrity than ever before. In the old days, you used to have a music career, or be on a TV show, and that has changed. Now you can get there through winning a reality show or being an online celebrity."

−Howard Bragman, publicist and author of Where's My Fifteen Minutes?

Our Disposable Culture Has Created Disposable Celebrities

We don't fix appliances anymore. We throw them out and get new ones. The same holds true for our celebrities. We're churning out disposable plasti-fame that's cheapening our culture. Reality TV is Exhibit A, granting attractive, quirky, hot-tempered, or even unstable people stardom for simply showing up on TV as themselves, with some careful behind-the-scenes glamorizing and staging of course. *The Real Housewives* phenomenon has become an instant-celebrity factory. For every genuine star produced by *American Idol,* we create a subset of mocked pseudostars whose primary purpose seems to be to get their names on everyone's lips even at the price of intense humiliation. Whatever did happen to Sanjaya Malakar, one of the finalists on *Idol's* Season 6, whose excruciating performances and wild hairdos created a firestorm of debate? Incensed that Sanjaya had not been eliminated, one female viewer went on camera and announced, "As a result of this I am going on a hunger strike. I am doing this because I believe that other talented contestants, who deserve a chance to win, are being eliminated because there are other people that think it would be funny to try and sabotage *American Idol* by voting for a lesser contestant."[2] Her hunger-strike announcement garnered hundreds of thousands of hits on YouTube.

Gandhi went on hunger strikes to protest British rule in India. Suffragettes endured hunger strikes in their fight for women's right to vote. And, in early twenty-first-century America, we have devolved to holding a hunger strike to protest a contestant on *American Idol*. Don't get me wrong. I am not humorless. I do find *Jersey Shore*'s Snooki and The Situation good for a chuckle. But where is our addiction to junk celebrity leading us as a culture?

It's leading us to what I call the Tila Tequila syndrome. Now you don't even need to audition for *American Idol* to become a celebrity. All you need to do is become a Twitter addict like Tila Tequila, whose incessant tweeting and wildly provocative, hypersexualized self-promotion garnered her millions of followers, crowned her the person with the most "friends" on MySpace.com in 2006, and landed her as number eight on *Forbes*'s Web Celeb 25 list, which purports to track "the biggest and brightest stars on the Internet, the people who have turned their passions into new media empires."[3] Her "empire building" included hosting a TV show where contestants stripped, hosting a bisexual reality dating show, writing a self-help book, producing songs and videos like "I Fucked the DJ" and "I Love U," where the phrase "I love you" is repeated over and over again to images of a very sexy Tila wielding a riding crop.[4] She also won Spike TV's annual Guys' Choice Award for "So Hot They're Famous" as well as Bravo's A-List Award for "A-List Drama Queen."[5]

You've got to hand it to Tila, considering she came out of nowhere in 2002 after being named Playboy.com's "Cyber Girl of the Week."[6] Her newest of many websites, TilasHotSpotDating.com, promises to be "the SICKEST dating site in the world." Tila calls her fans her "Tila Army Soldiers." It's an all-volunteer army comprised of celebrity addicts jonesing for a cheap fix from a super-hot, slightly demented genius for self-glorification. I actually have a perverse admiration for Tila and her ability to pull herself up by her G-string. It's her fans that I wonder and worry about. Why are so many people getting drunk on Tila Tequila?

The more available an addictive substance becomes, the easier it is to get hooked. As fast-food outlets and drive-thrus became ubiquitous, the number of food addicts skyrocketed in the United States. As prescription medications pervaded the culture, the number of pill heads soared. Similarly, as "celebrities" proliferate, accessible to us anytime via television or the Internet, the number of Americans obsessed with them is snowballing.

Out of the Mouths of Babes

Americans are getting hooked on celebrity at an ever-younger age. A perfect example is played out on YouTube as a three-year-old girl, Cody, has an emotional meltdown over teen heartthrob Justin Bieber. Her mom videotapes the scene.

Mom: Why are you crying?

Cody: Because I love Justin Bieber . . .

Mom: Why do you love Justin Bieber?

Cody: Because I know he loves me back . . .

Mom: Honey, we don't have to cry because we love Justin Bieber.

Cody (still crying): Yeah we do . . . sometimes . . .

Mom: What do you want Justin Bieber to do?

Cody: To be one of my family.

The video, which racked up more than 15 million views, comes to an end when the phone rings and the toddler smiles for the first time, saying, "I bet that's Justin Bieber!"[7] The innocent child articulates what adults secretly desire but are too embarrassed to say out loud. We want the celebrity to call us back. We want them to be part of our lives. And they are . . . in our fantasies.

We all desperately want to be near greatness. We want to be an original. But that's a scary place to go. So we let these genuine stars take the risks while we hang on for the ride.

Addiction Always Gets Down to Motive

The big question is: Why are we so interested in the celebrity? What's our motive? If it's because we respect their talent and enjoy their artistry, that's what I would consider healthy admiration. But if our obsession with the star is a form of escape, a way to numb ourselves, a vehicle to distract us from the pain and regret we feel about our own lives, then we are "using" the celebrity as a drug. And when we do that too often, we become addicted to the escape of focusing on their lives and not our own. Flipping though the gossip magazines while getting your nails done is one thing, but if you're fretting over Angelina Jolie's relationship with Brad Pitt, you've become a bit player in your own fantasy life.

The Celebrities We Love to Hate
Give Us the Biggest Pleasure Hit

Since the mission of my cable show *Issues* is to dissect topics average Americans talk about around the office water cooler, whatever they may be, I am constantly immersing myself in the smarmy details of the increasingly transparent personal lives of stars in trouble, be they A-list or D-list. I've covered Mel Gibson's racist rants and Lindsay Lohan's never-ending dramarama as she Ping-Ponged between court, jail, and rehab after a pair of DUIs.

July 6th, 2010, Issues

VELEZ-MITCHELL: The party is over for Lindsay Lohan. Today, judgment day. The troubled starlet broke down and wept. The party-hardy actress was at the center of a heated, furious hearing that dragged on all day long. Lilo boldly blew off the judge's very simple order: attend alcohol education classes once a week. Lindsay broke down and, tearfully sobbing, insisted she did everything she was told. Check out the waterworks on this one.

LINDSAY LOHAN, ACTRESS: I just wanted to take a minute to say that, you know, I—as far as I knew, I was being in compliant (sic) with my program. Having said that, I did do everything that I was told to do and did the best I could to, you know, balance jobs and showing up.

I'm sorry. I wasn't missing the classes just to—I wasn't doing anything like that. I was working mostly. I was working with children. It wasn't a vacation. It wasn't some sort of a joke. And I respect you and would take it seriously.

And I appreciate the program has done so much to help me finish early because I wanted to make sure that I would come back here making you happy and the court system and show that I meant everything I put into it. It's just been such a long haul, and I don't want—(Lindsay begins weeping) I don't want you to think that I don't respect you and your terms, because I really did think that I was doing what I was supposed to do. I mean that with all my heart.

VELEZ-MITCHELL: You've got to hand it to her. That was a performance of a lifetime! Luckily, the judge did not buy it.[8]

We soon learned that, during Lindsay's courtroom *tour de force*, she had "fuck you" written on her fingernails. "Lindsay Lohan's fingernail" quickly became the nation's number-one search item, sparking a *Washington Post* opinion piece headlined WHY IS AMERICA GOOGLING LINDSAY LOHAN'S FINGERNAIL? Good question.[9]

If only I devoted this much space in my brain to world history, I could be calling myself Dr. Velez-Mitchell by now. But I'm not the only one stuck in a celebrity time-suck vortex. At a time when an obscene amount of oil was spilling into the Gulf of Mexico, when obscene numbers of people were dying in Iraq and Afghanistan, when obscene numbers of children were living in makeshift tents in Haiti, why did America make Lindsay's obscene nails the top priority? Why is Lindsay Lohan a ratings bonanza?

The Real Cost of Cheap Celebrity Gossip

Let's face it. There are only so many hours in the day. We're already being inundated with and distracted by TV, Internet, cell phones, texting, e-mails, social networking, and so forth. The days of leisurely reading the newspaper from cover to cover are gone for most people. Our addiction to technology has shortened our attention span. Add to that an obsession with celebrity that has cheapened our intellectual priorities. My dad used to say, "Third-class minds talk about people, second-class minds talk about things, and first-class minds talk about ideas." While that's a sweeping generalization, there is something to be said for taking the time and mental effort to tackle complex, abstract ideas, be they of a philosophical or a scientific nature.

Time magazine, in a cover story on Thomas Edison, writes, "Inventors like Edison helped build America's unparalleled scientific and technological dominance, a dominance that, more than any

other single factor, made the 20th century the American century."
Time contrasts that with what is happening today. "American students seem to be losing interest in science. Only about one-third of
U.S. bachelor's degrees are in science or in engineering now, compared with 63% in Japan and 53% in China. "[10]

Clearly, there are many factors that contribute to this ominous
trend. But I think it's fair to ask: if we're focusing on trivial gossip,
do our minds lose the muscle to process difficult material? We've
reached the stage where people are more interested in voting for an
American Idol contestant than they are in voting for a member of
Congress. Whether it be Barack Obama or Sarah Palin, it seems the
few politicians who do inspire passion are precisely those who have
broken through to a superstardom that eclipses politics. They are
celebrities first, because in America today, it's personality first, policy
and principles second. That means image trumps ideas. In sobriety,
we say, "Principles before personalities." So, clearly, we are trapped
in an addictive mind-set.

Clearly, this mass psychosis of celebrity obsession is affecting the
national dialogue. Everybody seems to have a strong opinion about
Michael Jackson's death, John Edwards's love child, or Tiger's slew
of infidelities. It's a lot easier to master the facts of those stories than
it is to develop an opinion about . . . say . . . how to rescue the more
than 1 million Haitians displaced by the January 2010 earthquake.[11]
Could our obsession with celebrity be a form of self-medication
that ultimately undermines America's dominance as a culture?

Erratic, defiant, out-of-control celebs like Lindsay give us a
supercharged pleasure hit. Ditto for Mel Gibson. His infamous
insults against Jews, blacks, Latinos, gays, and women should've
made him persona non grata to most Americans by now. But we're
absolutely mesmerized by these superstar train wrecks. We get to

tell ourselves that maybe our mundane lives aren't so bad after all. *Look at Mel: he's handsome, rich, famous, powerful, and a great actor . . . and yet, he seems like a miserable, hateful human being. Look at Lindsay: she's beautiful, young, and famous . . . and yet, she seems like a lost soul. I guess my life's not so bad after all. I guess I'm grateful for what I have.*

"Everyone's dream is to be rich and famous. The biggest curse in someone's life is to be young, beautiful, and rich because there is only one place to go from there . . . down."

—Howard Samuels, Psy.D., licensed clinical psychologist, founder, and CEO of the Hills Treatment Center in Los Angeles

---

We Love to Watch Them Fall

We build stars up. We put them on a pedestal, and then we observe them as they become increasingly out of touch and start to assume that they're untouchable, that they "own Malibu" (to use Mel's phrase).[12] And then we wait . . . wait for them to slip and reveal their all-too-human character defects, be they alcoholism, drug addiction, sexual perversion, rage, or bigotry. Then we knock them down and crush them under our feet. *You're not such a big shot anymore, are you?* This is just how it is. It's human nature. Smart stars realize all this and understand that the price of fame and glory is living in front of a glass window with no curtains.

Today Celebs Have Nowhere to Run, Nowhere to Hide

As the number of celebrities has swelled, so have the number of media outlets reporting on them, further accelerating our obsession. From 2002 to 2005, I worked as a reporter for the nationally syndicated TV show *Celebrity Justice*, the granddaddy of these celebrity-focused media outlets. That show has now morphed into the wildly popular TMZ, which stands for Thirty Mile Zone, the theory being everything happens within a 30-mile zone in Hollywood. Harvey Levin, my dear friend and mentor, is the brainchild behind TMZ.com (and the TMZ TV show) and was also my boss at *Celebrity Justice*. Every morning at our 7:30 AM story meeting, Harvey would ask the same two questions: "Where's the celebrity?" and "Where's the justice?" That was the criteria for every story we did. When *Celebrity Justice* first started, plenty of skeptics actually wondered if we'd have enough material to fill a half hour every day. It quickly became apparent that Harvey was a visionary who grasped America's slide toward celebrity obsession just as the trend was about to take off and metastasize into mob madness.

Every Scandal Is a Cautionary Tale

As a journalist, I've always made it a point to scour these salacious scandals for socially relevant information. At *Celebrity Justice*, we went to great lengths to explain the serious legal issues underlying celebrity cases to give the viewers practical pointers about the law. That way, someone watching at home, perhaps contemplating divorce, can learn something useful watching a story about a nasty celebrity divorce. On my show *Issues*, I use these celebrity scandals as a springboard for sharing vital information about drug addiction, alcoholism, sex addiction, and codependency, issues which so often are at the heart of a star's disgrace. The phrase *Addict Nation* was a banner we frequently used on *Issues* long before it became the title of this book. In a perfect world, would I like to use all my television exposure to discuss solutions to the escalating and interrelated threats of pollution, global warming, overpopulation, world hunger, and overconsumption? Of course! And we do weave in those issues whenever we can. But my challenge is squeezing out useful knowledge from the stories that capture the popular imagination. Those are, increasingly, accounts of celebrities in hot water.

Tracking Troubled Stars Has Become an Industry Unto Itself

Our obsession with stars isn't just frittering away our time, it's clogging our court system. In a front-page story, the *New York Times* reported that, in one week in July 2010, "an army of government employees shooed Lindsay Lohan through a Beverly Hills courtroom to face jail for her latest probation violation. Meanwhile, a downtown jury gave Don Johnson $23.2 million for arrears on *Nash Bridges*, a judge let stand charges against Anna Nicole Smith's doctor, Jesse James fought a breach of contract claim, and Leif Garrett faced a heroin rap. Also, Ms. Lohan, in another Beverly Hills court, dealt with a suit over the emotional distress of someone she is accused of chasing" and "the Los Angeles County Sheriff's Department had acknowledged opening a domestic violence investigation involving Mel Gibson and the Russian model Oksana Grigorieva, with whom he has a child."[13] Movie stars, TV actors, and reality-show contestants are involved in controversy at a rate that's way out of proportion to their physical numbers. Drama and self-obsession are their stock and trade, and many of them appear to be working overtime. Call it professional deformation. On some very primitive, unconscious level, all attention is good.

"The narcissist goes around 'hunting and collecting' the way the expressions on people's faces change when they notice him. He places himself at the center of attention, or even as a figure of controversy. He constantly and recurrently pesters those near-est and dearest to him in a bid to reassure himself that he is not losing his fame, his magic touch, the attention of his social milieu."

—Dr. Sam Vaknin, author of Malignant Self Love[14]

Today Everyone with a Cell Phone Is a Potential Paparazzo

As part of their narcissism, many stars are convinced the rules do not apply to them. But technology has run headlong into elitism and crushed it. No longer can the famous have it both ways, enjoying all the privileges of celebrity with none of the restrictions. To a certain degree, stardom is a pact with the devil. Stars are showered with expensive bling, luxury-gift bags, VIP sections within VIP sections, and an overall defer-ence that would make a British royal blush. But the devil wants its due. Paparazzi packs roam Hollywood and Manhattan. Additionally, many stories are now broken by ordinary citizens who simply point a cell phone at a star who's misbehaving. Most cell phones record video and audio. If a celebrity acts out in public, there's a very good chance that, within minutes, the video of it will be posted on TMZ or competing sites. And, being human, stars have a tendency to forget that anything they say on a voicemail or to someone on the phone can be recorded. Mel Gibson's vicious, profanity-filled, racist, sexist telephone rant against his Russian supermodel baby mama was recorded by her and ended up on Radar Online, available for the whole world to hear. We could all judge for ourselves whether it was his unmistakable voice.

Are We Copycats of Their Bad Behavior?

As more of the famous turn infamous for ugly, self-centered, entitled, self-destructive, and illegal behavior, the dangerous message that
often comes through—to impressionable teenagers especially—is that
it's all somehow very glamorous. In his insightful book *The Mirror
Effect: How Celebrity Narcissism Is Seducing America,* Dr. Drew Pinsky
notes, "When stars are recorded indulging in high-risk behavior—
drinking heavily, taking drugs, refusing rehab, losing huge amounts of
weight in short amounts of time, making and releasing 'private' sex
videos—they are doing what psychological professionals consider
'modeling' that behavior: that is, broadcasting an image that serves as
a model for viewers of the broadcast."[15] I couldn't agree more. Millions of American teenagers are being inspired to behave in a boorish,
profane, overly sexualized, and even dangerous manner thanks to
these negative role models. That's why it's crucial to report on the consequences of celebrity misbehavior.

Stars Who Don't Slip Up
Become Our Gods and Goddesses

It cannot be easy for a major star to go through an entire career
without ever making the gossip columns for negative behavior. But a
surprising number of huge stars manage to keep their reputations
intact, despite today's aggressive, round-the-clock news cycle. Those
who manage to retain that aura of perfection become idolized, and
members of the herd can become "star struck"—literally intoxicated
by their object of affection.

One day, in West Hollywood, Julia Roberts apparently did something extraordinary. The *Pretty Woman* superstar is said to have
walked into a self-service yogurt shop. The *New York Post* reports,

"When she walked in alone, witnesses said, everyone was awestruck, silently gaping as she selected the mango flavor. 'The second she left, a man burst into tears and then bought mango just like Julia had,' said a source. 'Then he fished her napkin out of the trash.'"[16]

This man was clearly in the swoon of a superstar crush. In this case, the celebrity addiction manifests itself as a sick love. The obsessed fan deifies the star, putting them high up on a pedestal and prostrating himself before the famous person, as if to say, *I am nothing, and you are everything.*

We are pack animals. The need to have a leader of the pack is in our DNA. On a very primal level, we long to idolize someone we view as superior to us. The dictionary defines "venerate" as to regard "with heartfelt deference."[17] The need to honor is all about desire, the desire to love someone who seems supernaturally blessed with attributes like supreme beauty and talent. This innate desire to worship the "other," to bow down before that which is not ourselves, is instinctive.

It allows us to escape ourselves and let the tide of someone else's energy propel us. It allows us to lose ourselves and—for a few brief moments—experience the joy of free-falling through the cosmos. This need to surrender to that which is not ourselves is a basic human instinct. It's perfectly natural. However . . .

Addictions Occur When Our Natural Instincts Go Awry and Betray Us

Our natural instincts betray us when we fixate on someone who symbolizes something that is lacking in ourselves, be it beauty, fame, charisma, genius, or even something like sobriety. When I was a practicing drunk, with an out-of-control personal life, I developed a crush on someone who was sober and who lived a life of relative simplicity. I thought I desired that person as a lover, but I was subconsciously eroticizing my desire for the qualities and strength of character that individual possessed. Once I got sober and developed those same qualities myself, the crush evaporated. I had finally figured out how to personally embrace and express those same traits, so that the "other" person ceased to appear mystical and magical to me. But when the object of one's obsession is famous, it's generally impossible to develop the unique qualities that made that person a star.

It's a short leap from desiring to acquire the qualities someone else has to . . . desiring them, to stalking them. Remember that classic eighties' Calvin Klein fragrance ad? Between love and madness lies Obsession. How true is that?

Between Love and Madness

November 11, 2008, Los Angeles: Thirty-year-old Paula Goodspeed is found dead of an apparent suicide inside her car, which is parked near *American Idol* judge Paula Abdul's home. Along with prescription pills, cops find pictures of Abdul and the star's CDs. The license plate on the victim's car reportedly reads "ABL LV," presumably shorthand for Abdul Love. Abdul's photo dangles from the rearview mirror.[18]

It would turn out that Paula Goodspeed had made it on to *American Idol* back in 2005, getting to round three and singing before the judges. Simon Cowell actually remarked that he saw a "similarity" between Goodspeed and Adbul. Paula Abdul agreed, "I see it, definitely." "Really? I figure that's a compliment, because you're beautiful," Goodspeed replied to Abdul.

Goodspeed revealed to America that she had long been obsessed with the petite pop singer/dancer/choreographer. "I make life-size drawings of Paula. I've been drawing ever since I was a little kid, and my first drawing was of Paula Abdul."[19] Goodspeed described herself as a "fashion genius," but the infamously blunt *American Idol* panel did not agree. Simon Cowell latched on to the young woman's braces. "I don't think any artist on earth can sing with that much metal in your mouth anyway. You have so much metal in your mouth. That's like a bridge." A defiant Goodspeed vowed to continue to pursue a singing career. She later blogged about how hurtful the criticism was, but also posted a sexy photo of Paula Abdul on her MySpace page and wrote the caption. "My secret crush, shhhhhhh!!!!!!!!!"

This depressing story is an extreme example of what's happening to a lesser extent to millions of Americans. The ubiquity of celebrity has convinced millions of young Americans that they, too, are destined for fame. It's really setting people up for failure. Someone who is also psychologically and emotionally troubled is likely to wind up a dangerously obsessed fan.

"I think 20–25 percent of all kids believe they will be famous in their lifetime. A lot of kids don't even know what they want to be famous for. They just want to be famous. Twenty years ago, they all wanted their MBAs."

–Howard Bragman, *author of* Where's My Fifteen Minutes?

But What About ME?

Facebook, MySpace, YouTube, Twitter, and other social-networking sites have "tuned in" to our desire to be famous. I often hear people validate themselves, their projects, and even rate their prospective romantic partners according to how many times they pop up on the

Internet. In fact, if someone doesn't turn up on a Google search, they're often regarded with suspicion. Are they a fraud? It's as if the person doesn't exist.

We all know people who are hooked on self-promotion—constantly updating their "followers" and "friends" about every new development in their lives. Each clever tweet and video they post delivers a brief rush of adrenaline as the blogger presses send, and the possibility of finally becoming recognized for a special talent or unique contribution to the world is launched into cyberspace.

"There has been a big shift in terms of celebrity. It really has gone from your 15 minutes of fame to your fifteen seconds of fame. That is mostly attributed to the Internet. The Internet has made fame a lot more attainable to many people. That's why people's addiction or obsession with celebrity has increased. Because they think they can become famous a lot easier than before. Whether it be from making a funny video, or doing a prank, or crashing the White House."

—Perez Hilton, celebrity blogger

False Idols

Like all addiction, our fixation on celebrity is the result of spiritual bankruptcy. We are trying to fill a void within ourselves by either puffing ourselves up into something we're not or becoming obsessed with someone we consider above us. Ironically, this is a perversion of a desire for enlightenment and spiritual fulfillment.

When we are emotionally sober, we can revere "something greater than ourselves" in a number of healthy ways. Some might want to pray to their concept of God. Others may want to focus on their reverence for nature. Still others may aspire to learn from the life experiences of truly evolved individuals, like Mahatma Gandhi, Henry David Thoreau, Mother Teresa, and Martin Luther King Jr.

If we can take away one lesson from our culture's fixation on celebrity, it's that nobody is the center of the universe. A culture that puts some people on a pedestal is also telling other people that they don't count. We're all interconnected parts of a larger mosaic. Therefore, we should strive to treat everyone with the kindness and deference we now reserve for so-called VIPs.

As for becoming famous ourselves, when we humbly listen to our higher power, we will hear our true calling. That will lead us to do what we're really meant to do on this planet, whether it makes us famous . . . or not.

Chapter Five
THE PLAYERS: Addicted to Sex

J amie Jungers was a hot, hard-bodied, twenty-one-year-old nightclub hostess and lingerie model when she says Tiger Woods summoned her from across the room in a Las Vegas hangout. She says a
friend of the married superstar approached and informed her that
"TIGER WOODS" wanted to meet her. She immediately complied.
She says they drank, flirted, and spent the night together. "I was very
excited and honored that he was interested in me," Jungers told
Meredith Viera on *The Today Show*.[1] The ability to summon beautiful
women and to almost immediately bed them must have been an
exhilarating rush for Tiger—a man who'd grown up with the reputation of an overachieving geek. His nickname at college was Urkel, a
reference to an extremely nerdy character of the same name on the
TV show *Family Matters*.[2]

Because we covered the sexual shenanigans of Tiger Woods so
frequently on *Issues*, I earned the equivalent of a Ph.D. in this lurid
story, pouring over stacks of wire copy and magazine articles detail-
ing the stage names, dubious occupations, enhanced breast sizes,
tattoos, and private text messages of those involved with the case,
along with where and how they had their alleged sexual encounters
with the golf superstar. As graphic details continued to pour in from
emboldened ex-girlfriends who felt they had nothing to lose (and
possibly much to gain), the Tiger story exploded onto the national

consciousness, quickly turning into a classic case of Too Much Information.

Vanity Fair came out with an explosive article in which a bevy of women describe Tiger's "huge sexual appetite" in excruciatingly embarrassing detail. Did I really need to know that one of Tiger's estimated fourteen alleged mistresses claimed she told Tiger she didn't want to have sex (because she had her period), but he insisted she pull out her tampon anyway as he allegedly took her from behind in a church parking lot while, unbeknownst to them, a tabloid hack purportedly shot grainy photos of the tryst? Did I really need to know that a woman who runs an escort service claimed to *VF* that Tiger would pay up to $60,000 for a weekend with "college-cutie, girl-next-door types . . ."?

If half of what *Vanity Fair* laid out in that article is true, one could reasonably diagnose Tiger as a sex addict. That seemed the only explanation for Tiger's extraordinarily reckless actions . . . deeds that led to massive personal and professional wreckage. Even though Tiger remained coy, refusing to say what, specifically, he finally went into "treatment" for, we really didn't need to wait for this addict to self-diagnose. A drunk passed out in the gutter might never admit he's an alcoholic, though a sober passerby might casually look down and, in the flash of an eye, accurately identify him as a chronic boozer.

I tried to imagine how Tiger must have felt reading that lurid *Vanity Fair* article. In recovery, we talk about the "incomprehensible demoralization" of addiction. It's the blushing shame that the addict feels when he looks back remorsefully on his own behavior, wondering, *How did I become that person? Why did I feel compelled to do those things?*

"I had no control over my addiction—it was bigger than I was. Resistance was futile."

—Dave, recovering sex addict

It's the Intrigue That Hooks Us

One of the most fascinating aspects of sex addiction is that its "high" can be just as intoxicating as drugs or alcohol and is not primarily achieved by the sex act itself. While the addict may certainly derive pleasure from intercourse, oral sex, or any other type of physical sexual contact, it's the "dance" preceding the sex that drives the compulsion. That dance is known as "intrigue."

Most of us have experienced the enchanting exhilaration of falling in love. Most of us have been "under the influence" of romantic passion or lust at sometime in our life. There is nothing like it. It's the inspiration for spellbinding novels and heart-wrenching songs. More than almost anything else, it propels, inspires, and— yes—intoxicates us. Mother Nature made it that way.

The laws of "natural selection" dictate that women will seek to attract the strongest, healthiest, and most dependable man. She needs to know she can count on his support to raise healthy offspring and protect the family. For this reason, she is more likely to be choosy and less likely to have sex with every male who makes the offer. Men, on the other hand, have an innate yearning to "fertilize" as many females as possible. Just as a bee pollinates flowers, he will seek to plant his seed over and over again—sometimes to the point of obsession.

Addiction Is Instinct Gone Awry

With sex addicts, the instinct to pollinate has gone completely haywire. One sex therapist describes it as the "challenge to get partners to say OK . . . Sex addicts get a sense of 'job well done.'" So, when it comes to sex addiction, men seem, naturally, more vulnerable to the disease than women. Counselors report a large majority of the clients they treat for sex addiction are men.

"Boys are generally not made aware of, nor taught how to know or regulate their feeling states. Therefore, as men they struggle to know their interior experiences, and as a result frequently experience overwhelm. As testosterone is added to the mix, it is like gasoline on a fire. Behaviors of aggression, and impulsivity, including sexual impulsivity, all are enflamed."

—Gregory Guss, licensed clinical social worker

Bad Boys

Bad-boy biker Jesse James, who like Tiger also retreated to rehab, allegedly turned to as many as four mistresses. Why? Could it have been to compensate for what would appear to be a mushrooming sense of inadequacy in the face of the ever more astounding accomplishments of his very beautiful, very successful, very rich, very talented wife, actress Sandra Bullock? His sex scandal broke just days after Sandra picked up an Academy Award for best actress in *The Blind Side*, as Jesse sat in the audience looking up at her adoringly. Sandra must have felt blindsided by the women who came out of the woodwork. But in hindsight, the dynamic that led to the deceit seems clear. With an Oscar and a net worth estimated to be north of $80 million, Sandra had more than eclipsed her husband's fame as the host of the reality show *Monster Garage*, where he supervises mechanics as they soup up vehicles. It would seem that, while married to Sandra, his ego was often in need of a turbo charge.

How does an insecure man overcompensate for feelings of emasculation? By getting the approval of as many "other" women as possible. In the book *Sex and Love Addicts Anonymous*, the recovery program's founder sums up his sick, addictive relationships this way: "The objects of my passion were seen entirely in terms of their ability to fulfill my NEEDS . . . they were functions not human beings."[3]

In this case, the women seem to be everything his wife was not and would never want to be. Bullock is one of the most private, discreet actresses in Hollywood. Who did he allegedly have an affair with? Michelle "Bombshell" McGee, a heavily tattooed stripper with a penchant for posing in Nazi regalia who enjoys seminude karaoke. This brings us to another driving factor behind chronic infidelity. Remember Hugh Grant's fling with a sixty-dollar prostitute while he was dating Elizabeth Hurley, one of the world's most beautiful and elegant women? Yes, folks, we're talking about *that* syndrome, the Madonna/Whore syndrome, which is referenced in sex-addiction literature as a common symptom of sexually addictive behavior.

> "When you think about women who erotically dance and give a lap dance—the man sits there and the woman, who is naked or close to naked, gyrates around him, up and down him, as he sits there like a king on his throne."
>
> —*Alison Triessl, attorney and cofounder/CEO of Pasadena Recovery Center*

Secrets and Lies

The Madonna/Whore syndrome is a feature of the sex addict's "compartmentalization." That's a fancy term for living a double life, one with the angel, the other with the devil. That desire to possess both the good girl *and* the bad girl, along with the dueling impulses to be both the good boy *and* the bad boy, is a metaphor for the struggle all addicts face, over whether to follow the call of their higher yearnings or succumb to the lure of their baser instincts. It's light versus dark. It's integrity versus cynicism. It's sobriety versus addiction.

Medical experts estimate there are about 16 million sex addicts in the United States today (many of them undoubtedly fornicating as you read this).[4] Unfortunately, many Americans find it hard to believe that any of them—including Tiger or Jesse—really are sex addicts or that such a thing as sex addiction even exists!

"I am so sick of everybody claiming to be a sex addict when they get caught cheating," fumed a woman on a crowded couch at a party I attended. It was a Saturday night in April 2010. I was at a karaoke-themed birthday bash and had just wrapped up a room-clearing rendition of "Desperado" when an argument erupted among the few remaining party stragglers. The Tiger Woods cheating scandal had reached a deafening crescendo that week, and the seemingly endless media analysis was starting to grate on everyone's nerves. First Tiger and then Jesse had reacted to their unmasking by running off into rehab (presumably for sex addiction). Many, if not most, people saw it as a cowardly cop-out. "It's such a ridiculous excuse," someone else yelled. "These guys are just cheaters and horn-dogs, not addicts!" Comedian and HBO host Bill Maher also pushed the notion of sex addiction being a joke with a New Rule: *"Stop saying 'sex addict' like it's a bad thing!"* And *"You want to know the surest way that you can spot a 'sex addict'? He's got a penis."*[5]

Personal accountability is important to people. The public gets annoyed when depraved celebrities try to patch up every monstrous misstep with a recovery meeting. Sex addiction is viewed as a get-out-of-jail free card for men who are merely lustful cads and liars. While people have no trouble accepting alcoholism, drug addiction, and even food addiction, a lot of Americans simply refuse to buy the notion that someone can become a sex junkie. To date, sex addiction is not listed as an official "disorder" in the American Psychiatric Association's diagnostic manual.[6] Hopefully, that will change.

In the groundbreaking book, *Sex and Love Addicts Anonymous,* the unnamed man who founded the recovery program that bears that name says he, too, was greeted with hostility and skepticism when he began to share his experiences as one of the first self-acknowledged sex addicts back in the 1970s. "Others could not understand my suffering . . . Even as I described the pain brought by these addictive patterns of compulsive sexual activity and emotional intrigue, these people complained that their lives did not contain 'enough' of this. They could not seem to understand that . . . insanity is *insanity* regardless of whether it is encountered in drinking or romance!"[7]

Since all addiction can be described as an overpowering craving to repeatedly engage in an activity that provides temporary relief at the expense of terrible consequences, sex addiction can be defined as an uncontrollable impulse to have sex despite dire consequences to family, friends, and community, and to one's own self-esteem.

"At the time there is an incredible adrenaline rush . . . it's a connection that I found I couldn't replicate anywhere else. But immediately after that experience is over, I mean driving back home, there is this incredible letdown and you're just in a wash of shame . . . I was trying to get nonsexual needs met sexually, and that was the only way I knew how to meet those needs."

—Female sex addict, Dateline NBC, *February 24, 2004*[8]

They key phrase in the above quote is "trying to get nonsexual needs met sexually." To say that sex addicts have sex for the wrong reasons is a monumental understatement. The addict often uses sex to escape from painful feelings of worthlessness and alienation by reassuring themselves of their value through repeated conquests. For men especially, who account for about two-thirds of the sex addicts in the United States, to "score" is to achieve "success," which is to be a "winner." The terrible irony is that the sex addict so cheapens the act of sex with these base motivations that he gradually *robs himself* of his dignity and integrity. As the addiction progresses, the feelings of worthlessness increase.

There is another irony to sex addiction. While the act of sex is, theoretically, about intimacy, the sex addict is terrified of intimacy. He feels much more secure in using sex for the thrill of conquest, for self-validation, to escape painful feelings, for revenge, or to outwit a rival. Sometimes a sex addict will add a new partner as "insurance," in case one of his other sex partners slips away. For the sex addict, any manipulative reason to have sex is preferable to the purest motivation . . . to express love.

"Men love sex and men say, 'We think about sex all the time and there is nothing wrong with thinking about sex all the time.' And they are probably right. But when having sex, watching sex, having multiple partners takes over your life to the point where you cannot function . . . where you spend eight hours in front of a computer . . . where days and nights pass and you don't even know what day or time it is, then it has literally taken over your life."

—Alison Triessl, attorney and cofounder/CEO of Pasadena Recovery Center

---

A Double Life Requires Secrets and Lies

Secrets will reveal themselves unless they're protected! The way you protect secrets is with lies. Case in point, presidential wannabe John Edwards. The former North Carolina senator's sexual obsession with a woman who was not his cancer-stricken wife, while he was on the campaign trail, resulted in a love child, which was a BIG SECRET that needed to be protected with BIG LIES. What already had the makings of a tawdry sex scandal morphed into something much more shameful as Edwards's long-time aide Andrew Young came forward claiming the candidate begged him to lie for him and say the child was his, even though Young was married with children of his own. Says Young, "He was one of my best friends, we jogged together, our kids played together." Young says he reluctantly agreed to play daddy in the charade.

It would be more than two years before John Edwards would finally come clean and tell the world *he* was, in fact, the father. But in that time, Edwards repeatedly lied on camera, claiming it was impossible for him to be the father because of the timing of the child's birth. Edwards insisted, before the nation, that the affair was long over at the time the baby girl was conceived. The extent and complexity of John Edwards's lies stunned even hardened politicians and journalists who thought they had seen it all. But when viewed through the prism of addiction, it's really not that shocking at all.

Lying Is How Addiction Comes Packaged

While John Edwards, to my knowledge, never checked himself into rehab, to me he clearly appears to be, at the very least, a love addict. A close cousin of sex addiction is addiction to love and/or romance. Undoubtedly, John Edwards romanticized his cheating and lying and justified it as what he needed to do "for love." Unlike Tiger Woods, who appears to have played a numbers game, adding up conquests the way he racked up golf majors titles, John Edwards probably regarded himself as being in the throes of a passionate "love affair" that was so intense he risked everything.

Two hallmarks of love and/or romance addiction are grandiosity and drama. When Edwards teamed up with his mistress, Rielle Hunter, the pair whipped up a staggering display of both. His obsessive relationship with this woman he met on a street corner destroyed his political career, his marriage, and his reputation and branded him as a serial liar, a cheat, and a cad the world over.[9]

Healthy Versus Sick Love

How do we distinguish between addictive love patterns and healthy ones? I would define healthy love as being grounded in self-love, which is totally different from narcissism. If you love and respect yourself, if you have integrity, dignity, and autonomy, then you don't need to *use* a love relationship to bolster your fragile ego, or indeed *use* it for any purpose. It just is. Healthy love involves sharing yourself, exposing your core being, communicating with your lover, and supporting him or her as a life partner with *no* ulterior motives. Easier said than done.

In addictive love, the lover is used as a *tool* to achieve goals, enhance self-image, or solve internal problems. The act of love becomes a *portal* to escape, just like a drug. This is something I've seen myself do over and over again and just recently, after researching this subject, was able to see this pattern objectively and put it into words. For example, I've often felt an enhanced sense of self-esteem when I was seen out with a very attractive lover. Beauty is fantastic! But when you "use" your partner's beauty for your own purposes, as opposed to simply celebrating that beauty for what it is, then you are engaging in an addictive love pattern. Being obsessed with your lover's looks (or your own) might even be described as a *beauty blackout*! Addicts are often desperate to stuff painful internal issues and will sometimes compensate for their inner turmoil by making everything look perfect on the outside.

"Our brains have the ability to manufacture their own chemical 'hits,' which are just as addicting as ingested substances, perhaps even more so."

—Dave, recovering sex addict

Risky Behavior Enhances the Love Addict's High

One big reason love and sex addicts create so much drama and practice risky behavior is that all that excitement enhances the high. In short, the addictive lover uses the relationship like a bottle of booze or a pill. In *Is It Love or Is It Addiction?*, psychologist and addiction specialist Brenda Schaeffer writes, "It has now been confirmed that the rush of intoxication is associated with the neurological release of endorphins and many other mood elevators . . . In addictive love, we unconsciously use the objects of love, sex, or romance to stimulate the chemicals in the brain to produce the high . . . we arouse ourselves with the excitement, fear, rage, or melodrama that exemplify addictive love."[10] In this respect, it appears John Edwards was on a bender.

The shocking sex scandal reached a crescendo when word broke that a *sex tape* allegedly existed, purportedly involving John Edwards and Rielle Hunter. The Washington beltway gasped, along with the rest of the country. Who in their right mind would even think about making a sex tape with their secret mistress when they were married with children and trying to become president of the United States? The only answer I can think of is: a love addict, or a pair of love addicts. What a nifty way to ratchet up the endorphin-producing excitement, fear, and dramarama the love addict craves.

Romance Versus Recklessness

Our culture indoctrinates us to become love and romance addicts. It's what sells movie tickets and the books we read around the swimming pool. Love addicts have a compulsion to romanticize ordinary situations, seeking out fairy-tale story lines by embellishing mundane reality with fantasy, which creates the rush. For women, a common fantasy is being rescued by a strong man who will become their champion and magically solve all their problems. What did Rielle Hunter tell *GQ* magazine in her sit-down to discuss her relationship with "Johnny"? "I had this thing in my head like a lot of women, where you want your man to stand up on a cliff and scream 'I LOVE HER.' You know, the knight in shining armor."[11] That was the fantasy. The reality was her scandal-plagued lover, Johnny, was married and going on national television trying to smooth it over by telling the American people there was only one woman he ever loved, his wife, Elizabeth. Rielle says after one such pronouncement John called her to apologize, allegedly adding, "It doesn't mean anything." Again, the split-screen life, maintained through lies, is such a hallmark of addiction. And it creates so much wreckage.

Sometimes I look at these scandals and try to give the participants the benefit of the doubt, wondering, *Hey, it's messy love, but could it still be love?* Why can't addictive love or addictive sex be compatible with true love? Because you can't express truth while swimming in a sea of lies! At the heart of profound love is truth, sharing with someone else the truth of who you are, opening up, revealing, becoming vulnerable, letting the "other" see you without a filter. Deception, by definition, means hiding, misrepresenting, building walls, and presenting falsehood as truth. Lying kills intimacy because at the moment you should be sharing, you're withholding. When lying is a way of life, it destroys your ability to really love anyone.

With Almost All Addicts, Lying Is a Way of Life

Tiger Woods's deception increased exponentially as his cheating—and his apparent disease of sex addiction—progressed. It would seem he was not just lying to his wife, but also to his alleged mistresses and to the public. Days before his sex scandal broke, the superstar father of two young children was asked by a TV interviewer, "Family first and golf second. Always be like that?" "Always," Tiger replied, essentially lying to a global audience.[12]

As a bevy of waitresses, strippers, swimsuit models, nightclub hostesses, and porn stars came forward claiming to have slept with Tiger, some of the alleged mistresses expressed shock, saying they thought they were the *only* mistress with whom he was cheating on his wife. A porn star who goes by the name Joslyn James released a slew of X-rated text messages in a bid to prove her claim that she had a three-year relationship with Tiger, during which time she insists she was convinced she was the only "other" other woman. While she may be guilty of naiveté, Tiger's alleged behavior took "compartmentalization" to new depths. He masterfully kept each woman ignorant of the others as if they were toys to be put in separate drawers. It was a *tour de force* of organization . . . until the toys came to life.

Rationalizations "R" Us

Addiction becomes the dictator of the mind, body, and soul, the authoritative voice that commands the addict as a dictator would his slave. The commands go through the addict's mind and come out as rationalizations. Addicts are the most superb rationalizers because they constantly practice at justifying bizarre and outrageous behavior.

When Tiger Woods emerged back on the world stage after more than a month in rehab, he gave the following speech.

Tiger Woods, Press Statement, February 19, 2010

"I knew my actions were wrong, but I convinced myself that normal rules didn't apply. I never thought about who I was hurting. Instead, I thought only of myself. I ran straight through the boundaries that a married couple should live by. I thought I could get away with whatever I wanted to. I felt that I had worked hard my entire life and deserved to enjoy all the temptations around me. I felt I was entitled."

In one breath, Tiger listed many of the key themes surrounding addictive behavior: a sense of entitlement, a sense of being different, a sense that the normal rules don't apply, which twelve-step programs call "terminally unique," and a disrespect for the boundaries of conventional behavior.

A Key Tenet of Recovery Is Making Amends, Apologizing

In recovery we don't just apologize when it's convenient to do so, but—especially—when it's inconvenient. We also don't withhold apologies because we feel that person has also hurt us or is somehow unworthy. Making amends is one of the most powerful steps in sobriety because it allows us to reconnect with another person, shed our painful guilt, and begin anew with a clean slate. It's all about taking responsibility for "our" actions and keeping our side of the street clean. It really doesn't matter what the other person did or who he or she is.

Several of Tiger's alleged mistresses insist they really believed they were in a serious relationship with Woods and—in the wake of revelations of an avalanche of sexual indiscretions—say they, too, feel betrayed. Some have wept on national television. X-rated film star Joslyn James demanded an apology from Woods.

> "He saw her several times each month for three years. He sent her over 1,000 texts. He told her, 'The great thing is, we have a lifetime of this,' and 'You please me more than anyone ever has or ever will.' . . . He needs to apologize because he told her that he loved her, that he was only with her and his wife, that there was no one else. . . . She's not like a used Coke can that some people throw out their window as they're driving along like, 'OK, let's just forget about that.' No, this is a human being that has feelings."
>
> *—Gloria Allred, attorney for Joslyn James*
> *(aka Veronica Siwik-Daniels) on* Issues, *February 19, 2010*[13]

These women may be what cynics describe as "low-hanging fruit," the easy prey of a rich and famous man, but so what? Tiger apologized to his wife, his children, his fans, and even fellow golfers. Why not apologize if you've been intimate with someone under false pretenses and they feel hurt? Tiger's apparent refusal to say "I'm sorry" to these alleged mistresses speaks to his continuing objectification of these women, his treatment of them as factotums who were there to serve a function. But he's not alone. Despite all the advances women have made, misogyny is still rampant in America. You might even say sexism is a cultural addiction all its own. Today, most Americans continue to favor one gender over the other despite the hurtful or damaging effects on the society as a whole.

America's Porn Habit

There has been a sea change in our culture in the last quarter of a century. One difference? Pornography. Pornography exploded when VCRs arrived in the late 1970s, allowing consumers to take it home and watch it without the fear of being observed by a neighbor or colleague. "The first thing that a lot of people did when they got their VCR was rent or purchase an adult movie. *Deep Throat. Devil in Miss Jones. Behind the Green Door. Debbie Does Dallas.* That's what they asked for," a porn-industry trade magazine publisher told *60 Minutes*, adding that, until the advent of home video players, "most people had never seen an adult movie, because they had to go out in public, to a theater, to see it."[14]

Although statistics in the porn arena can be unreliable, given the shady nature of the biz, it's estimated that—today—Hollywood releases something like 11,000 pornos a year—nearly twenty times the number of mainstream movies released in theaters.[15]

Porn's popularity went into the stratosphere with the arrival of the Internet, which made graphic sex available with the click of a mouse. It is widely reported that more than 70 percent of men in the eighteen to thirty-four age bracket visit a pornographic site in a typical month.[16] Don't believe it? Just Google the word "porn." One hundred fifty *million* links will pop up.

It seems all of corporate America wants to "penetrate" this market. Most of the big hotel chains offer X-rated films on in-room pay-per-view television systems. Adult films are bought by a whopping 50 percent of their guests, accounting for nearly 70 percent of hotel in-room profits. These are, for the most part, businessmen on business trips, average guys.[17]

The nation's largest satellite/cable companies make hundreds of millions of dollars each year from adult programming, distributing sexually explicit material to their customers, although it's been noted that the word "porn" doesn't pop up in their annual reports. Americans now spend more than $10 billion a year on adult entertainment, which is as much as they spend attending sports events, music, or mainstream movies.[18]

The consumers of Internet and video porn are, overwhelmingly, someone's husband, boyfriend, and/or father. Of course, it almost goes without saying but . . . the vast majority of porn consumers are men whose wives or girlfriends have *no idea* their men are hooked on porn! We'd all prefer to live in the delusion that graphic porn is being bought by "that weird guy next door."

"There are so many wonderful things about the Internet, but one thing that is not so wonderful is that people have been able to really isolate, go into their home, and for years now just get on the computer all day every day and build up these sexual urges and desires."

*—Alison Triessl, attoney and cofounder/
CEO of Pasadena Recovery Center*

How many American men are keeping their porn-viewing habits secret from their wives and girlfriends, sneaking onto the computer when she's asleep or out? Lots! Tens of millions of men are forsaking true intimacy with their partner and opting instead for the quick and easy high offered by hard-core Internet porn.

Porn and Crack, Nothing Else Can Compete

Like crack cocaine, porn is highly addictive. Porn watchers can quickly develop a dependency on images of explicit sexual activity that often make their real life relationships seem dull or, even worse, irrelevant. Not many flesh-and-blood females can compete with the imagery that's available at the touch of a button today. There's no need to wine and dine a virtual Internet sex object. You don't even need to shave or bathe.

In stark counterpoint to the lazy passivity of the viewer is the grotesque and extreme physicality of the "actors" participating. "Most girls who enter this industry do one video and quit. The experience is so painful, horrifying, embarrassing, humiliating for them that they never do it again," says a prominent porn-industry media observer.[19] The kind of sex women are required to perform in porn is precisely the kind of sex many, if not most, women are loathe to perform in real life: being penetrated by two men at once, anal sex, humiliation, and acting out rape fantasies, etc., etc., etc.

> "I guess I see pornography in our society as a . . . perversion of sexuality. It removes the 'human' from the experience. As an addict, I used people to feed my fantasies, which I believed would bring me comfort. I did not see people as they were; I saw only my own distorted image of how they could bring me pleasure."
>
> —*Dave, recovering sex addict*

Addiction is a progressive disease, and that holds true for cultural addictions. In one century, we've gone from men becoming sexually excited by the sight of an ankle to many men requiring graphic sexual imagery on a giant high-definition plasma screen in order to experience arousal.

A High Tolerance for Smut

As we've discussed, addicts invariably spiral downward because they build up a tolerance for their substance of choice and need

ever-increasing amounts of it to achieve the same high. This principle applies to behavioral habits like sex and porn addiction. A man
who gets hooked on porn often finds himself needing ever more
graphic imagery to "get off." It's not long before vanilla sex barely
registers. Therefore, he will need porn playing on the bedroom TV
screen to "enhance" his experience with a flesh-and-blood woman.
Porn also fosters a sexist outlook that can carry over into everyday
interactions by indoctrinating the porn consumer to perceive
women as sexual objects and commodities to use or abuse at his
whim.

"Most pornographic material portrays women as subservient
and slaves to men. So they (male porn consumers) have a
major problem relating to women in any type of normal social
setting because their idea of a woman is so skewed by what
they see in pornography."

—Alison Triessl, attorney and cofounder/CEO
of Pasadena Recovery Center

Many women feel they're in a losing battle to mimic the shape of
a porn-star body that is often surgically enhanced to turn on a man.
As the obesity-crisis escalates, with two-thirds of Americans overweight or obese, the hour-glass-figured woman who pops up in
adult films has become even more of a precious commodity.

If the proliferation of porn continues unabated, we could be
headed toward a future of loneliness where cyberporn is the primary
way in which we experience sexual arousal and gratification. Picture
a world where a human touch and the exchange of human fluids
is considered horribly old-fashioned or even dirty. In the 1993
futuristic dystopian action film *Demolition Man*, the two leads,
Sylvester Stallone and Sandra Bullock, engage in a safe and "touch

free" virtual intercourse by wearing sex simulators mounted on their heads. On some level, it seems we have already arrived.

We Need Some Old-Fashioned Feminism

Don't get me wrong. I'm not a prude. I've seen highly erotic films that include nudity, and some of them were pretty darn entertaining. There's even a soft-core subgenre where romantic story lines, beautiful actors, and gorgeous backdrops elevate the material to the point where it's still an adult movie, but it's not smut. And there are also films that touch on taboo fetishes, like dominance and submission, that are handled with an artful sense of playfulness or experimentation that redeem the material, be it a remake of *The Story of O* or *Lady Chatterley's Lover*. Sometimes, in these films, the sex is simulated and sometimes it's real. That's not how I draw the line. Where does it cross over into denigration, thereby becoming something morally objectionable? In 1964, Supreme Court Justice Potter Stewart tried to define "hard-core" pornography by famously explaining, "I know it when I see it."

If what I am watching is highly graphic, demeaning, and/or violent porn where the theme and imagery is the violation and denigration of women, I object to it on a visceral level. Many women probably feel the same way, but in an effort to appear cool, worldly, and open-minded, they have embraced the porn habits of their significant others or concluded that it's just a nasty habit that they're going to have to put up with, like the boxer shorts he leaves on the bedroom floor. Porn is a lot more pernicious than dirty underwear. While hard-core porn denigrates all participants by prostituting what is meant to be the most private and personal of human interactions, let's be real, it demeans women more. Maybe the male actors don't really care that they are being exploited as well because at least they are in the throes of arousal. An aroused male is a male experiencing pleasure. Since he's experiencing pleasure, his exploitation is less acute than the female, who is on the receiving end and who may be feigning pleasure as called for by the director.

There's another key reason why hard-core porn is so horribly exploitive to the point of being dangerous. Addiction is progressive, meaning it invariably gets more extreme. As the porn consumer becomes increasingly deadened to the material, requiring ever more graphic material for stimulation, he will often stray into pornography that involves extreme violence. There are dozens of subgenres of hard-core porn that involve sadistic torture and practices too X-rated to mention here. There's even "amputee porn." There are crush films, where helpless small animals are crushed to death, which apparently creates arousal in some very sick minds. And, as we know, although thankfully I've never seen one, snuff films exist where women are actually murdered on tape in the course of a sexual act. And then there's . . . child porn.

Hooked on Kiddie Porn

In 2009, a United Nations expert estimated there are more than 4 million websites worldwide that contain images of child porn, 4 million . . . and growing! And, says the expert, the images on those sites are becoming increasingly graphic. There are numerous examples of how an addiction to violent porn or child porn has resulted in the addict becoming obsessed with acting out the sick, forbidden act *in real life*! Violent pornography may not be the cause of sex crime, but it is often found at the scene.

One sunny day in October 2009, seven-year-old Somer Thompson was walking home from school in Orange Park, Florida, with her brother and sister when she decided to run ahead of them. The adorable little girl was never seen alive again. Two days later, her body turned up in a Georgia landfill. After a lengthy investigation, Jarred Harrell, a twenty-four-year-old neighbor, was arrested and charged with her murder.

It would turn out that, back in August 2009, two months *before* little Somer was defiled and murdered, the suspect's roommates had gone to the police about him.[20] They had told cops they'd looked into his computer and discovered a slew of graphic child pornography that included a file named "toddler insertion."[21] The roommates were so freaked out they handed Harrell's computer to the cops and begged them to do something. Apparently, law enforcement didn't regard it as the critical, time-sensitive matter it would turn out to be. Authorities took months to complete the forensic examination of the computer. By the time they wrapped up their work and arrested Harrell, little Somer was long dead. The arrest warrant affidavit says, as part of their investigation, cops found "a video and multiple still images of a partially nude white female child between the ages of 3 to 5 years old. The defendant was . . . seen on the recording taking his hand and spreading the child's buttocks to expose her rectum and vagina."[22] Cops believe Harrell molested and videotaped this unnamed child long before he allegedly attacked and murdered little Somer Thompson.

After they finally connected the dots and charged Harrell with Somer's murder, reporters asked cops why they dragged their feet and failed to make a timely arrest of Harrell, given the child porn in the computer his roommates had dropped in their laps months earlier. The implication was clear. Had cops arrested him quickly, on kiddie porn charges, he would have been behind bars and not walking the streets free to allegedly act out his sick fantasies on an innocent little girl. The sheriff defended himself by saying that plenty of men who watch child porn don't act on it.

Issues on HLN, March 26, 2010

SHERIFF RICK BESELER, CLAY COUNTY: Not everyone who . . . who participates in that type of conduct actually ever becomes an offender that attacks someone. Mr. Harrell had not come onto anyone's radar screen as far as someone who might commit a crime like this. The things that he was accused of early on, you know, don't necessarily . . . not necessarily a precursor to this type of event.

VELEZ-MITCHELL: Well, really, Sheriff? We have to ask. Take a look at the affidavit for Harrell's arrest from last month, describing the videos cops were given back in August in this computer. There were twenty-four pornographic images of children and five movies that contained child pornography. [23]

ALISON TRIESSL, DEFENSE ATTORNEY/ADDICTION SPECIALIST: Yes, there's a bit of a leap that this person would go out and kill somebody, but they should have been on the radar looking at this person, interviewing him immediately, taking him in, questioning him. More . . . much more could have been done.

VELEZ-MITCHELL: Any thoughts, Samuel?

SAMUEL THOMPSON: (Somer's father): Well, that's . . . that's some pretty heavy information there.[24]

Addicts are ticking time bombs. It's only a matter of time before they implode and destroy their own lives . . . or explode in an act of violence against someone else. While it's true that, statistically, only a tiny percentage of hard-core porn watchers will act out those images in real life, it's a good bet that those men who *are caught* acting out sick, violent sexual fantasies on an unwilling female or child are extremely likely to be heavy porn users and/or compulsively trolling the Internet for sex. While these violence-prone men may be sociopaths or have some even more pronounced mental illness, there is often an addictive component to their dysfunction. Yet, usually, society labels them as violent psychotics without adding the *addict factor* into the equation.

The hit *Dateline NBC* show *To Catch a Predator* dramatically proves that the mental image we have of a sex offender is in sharp contrast with the reality. These men are not hobos in frayed trench coats who've crawled out of some gutter. They are average Joes from all walks of life—teachers, doctors, servicemen, men of the cloth—caught using the Internet to arrange sex with underage girls or boys.

Many of these men are married. Many have girlfriends. These women generally have no clue about the true sexual proclivities and inclinations of the men they are with. *They are living with a stranger who keeps the most personal part of his life a total secret!*

When Boston's infamous "Craigslist Killer" Philip Markoff was arrested and charged with the murder of a masseuse, his fiancé initially defended him, unable to fathom that her preppy, medical student boyfriend had a secret life that was 180 degrees shy of her perception of him. Then cops found several pairs of women's panties under the bed they shared, along with dozens of plastic flex-cuff restraints, plus a hollowed-out copy of *Gray's Anatomy* containing a gun believed to be the murder weapon.[25] Markoff accessed his secret world through Craigslist and other sites, where he would troll for strippers, escorts, and, some reports claim, transvestites. *48 Hours/Mystery* reports investigators believe one of Markoff's e-mail addresses was "sexaddict5385."[26] Before he could go to trial for murder, Markoff committed suicide in his jail cell, leaving his former fiancé's name scrawled in blood on the wall. These are extreme examples of what is happening all over America.

Addiction operates best behind a cloak of secrecy. Just as an alcoholic hides the bottle in the medicine closet, those addicted to porn, and those with unusual fetishes, often keep these impulses hidden from the one person who should know about them, their spouse or significant other. Consequently, the secret behavior festers and grows and takes on a life of its own as the addict's primary relationship is eclipsed and becomes increasingly superficial and empty.

Let's Get Honest About Sex

One of the tenets of recovery is "rigorous honesty." We keep secrets and tell lies to cover up sexual urges because our culture is intolerant of genuine, natural, unscripted human sexuality. In a more evolved society, we would embrace our inborn sexual urges and discard primitive taboos and pointless shame. Instead, we wage "campaigns" against sexuality. Often, those shouting the loudest—from the pulpit or the podium—are secretly addicted to the very thing they're denouncing. Psychiatrists call this *reaction formation*, where you condemn the very thing that secretly obsesses you for two reasons: to convince yourself that you don't want it and to create a smokescreen so others don't figure out you want it!

Sexuality is one of the most incredible aspects of the human experience. Most want to believe it is a spiritual, beautiful part of life. We need to encourage our lawmakers, teachers, and political leaders to stop treating sexuality like it's a crime. When we tell people sex is intrinsically "bad," they equate it with evil and express it as such. We have demonized sex as a culture, and we're paying the price in the form of sexual abuse and sexual crime. Let's get honest about what sex and love are really like! Homosexuality, fetishes,

sexual games, power exchanges, open relationships, bisexuality—
these are just some of the lifestyles and natural sexual activities we
should openly acknowledge and accept so they are not forced into
shameful secrecy or expressed pornographically.

I should know. It took me decades to come to terms with my own
homosexuality in order to conform to a society that told me there
was something wrong with those innate desires. So I went into
denial about my feelings toward members of the same sex and proceeded to become an alcoholic to drown the sadness and confusion
that wouldn't go away. When I finally sobered up more than fifteen
years ago, I could lie to myself no longer. Eventually, the truth came
out as it always does.

Toxic secrets will either implode, destroying the secret keeper, or
explode in violence against an innocent. There is another way.
Acceptance. It seems like an easy call.

Chapter Six
THE BLOODLUSTERS: Addicted to Crime

D ecember 27, 2009, two days after Christmas. A toned, twenty-three-year-old graduate student moves briskly past her parents' ornately decorated tree as she heads out for a run. Candice Moncayo is an attractive brunette who has the bearing of an athlete. She's studied martial arts since childhood and is a long-distance runner. Though home for the holidays, Candice has the discipline to keep to her exercise schedule. She moves at a good clip as she jogs down the streets of this well-manicured suburb outside San Diego. It's a gorgeous day, so much warmer than the Colorado weather she's learned to endure. It feels good to be home in the California sunshine. She heads into a community park where jogging trails run alongside a shimmering lake.

Candice is almost at the end of her eight-mile run when she sees a tall, bulky man with a crew cut and blue jeans coming from the other direction. "Good morning," she says cheerfully as she breezes past him. A millisecond later, Candice feels his considerable weight slamming into her. He tackles her to the ground. Candice lets out a piercing scream. "Shut up!" he says, leaning over her. *He's going to rape me,* she thinks, terrified. "You're going to have to kill me first," she cries. "That can be arranged," is his reply. Her thumping heart feels like it's going to fly out of her chest. The bulky, six-foot-two attacker grabs Candice by the shoulders, shaking her violently.

Candice senses it's a life or death moment. Suddenly she remembers a martial arts move she's practiced since childhood and forcefully elbows the man in the nose. He's hurt and momentarily releases her. She jumps up and runs like hell, faster than she's ever run before. She reports the crime to police.

Two months later, Thursday, February 25, 2010. It's the same suburb outside San Diego. At the local high school, class lets out for the day. A seventeen-year-old senior, with blue eyes and dirty blonde hair, hops into her BMW. Blessed with homecoming-queen looks, Chelsea King is also a straight-A student who has already been accepted into several colleges. On top of tutoring other students and playing French horn for the San Diego Youth Symphony, she's also a member of the cross-country team. An overachiever, she finds running is a great way to burn off stress. It's a perfect day for a run. Chelsea pulls her car into the local community park's lot and heads out onto the trails that wind alongside that same shimmering lake. She is never seen alive again.

Chelsea didn't have to die. We could have prevented it. Why didn't we?

In the days following Chelsea's disappearance, a small army converges on the park. Hundreds of law-enforcement and volunteer searchers comb the brush around the lake. The atmosphere is somber and yet electric. Teams of divers navigate the murky waters. Helicopters circle overhead. Police dogs sniff for a trace of the victim. News trucks set up, raising their masts to the heavens. Neighbors are interviewed. The sheriff's department holds news conferences. Cable hosts, including myself, pour over the clues. *Where did she go? How do we solve the mystery?* By now, we are all familiar with how this morbid ritual unfolds from the moment the yellow crime-scene tape is unrolled.

Chelsea's gut-wrenching case has all the classic conventions.

Soon comes an unnerving discovery. Chelsea's underwear is spotted in the brush with what appears to be semen on it. The DNA is run against a computer database of sex offenders. A name comes back. Cops arrest John Gardner III as he walks out of a local restaurant. He's a thirty-year-old, 230-pound white male with a crew cut who looks like a linebacker. Cops show his mug shot to the first jogger, Candice Montoya. "Yep, he's the same guy," she tells them. Cops believe this sex predator turned this scenic park into his personal hunting ground.

It turns out John Gardner had been staying with his mother, just an easy walk from where the attacks occurred. Neighbors didn't have any idea this registered sex offender was living in their midst. In the sex-offender registry, Gardner's listed address is in another town two hours away.

As I prepare my research for the night's show, I can't believe how easily John Gardner made a mockery of California's sex offender registry. We can track FedEx packages across the country and know where they are every minute of the day, but we can't track a 230-pound lug, who's a registered sex offender, from town to town in Southern California?

It doesn't take much research to figure out that Gardner's case is typical. Nationally, about one in seven sex offenders are not properly listed in the registry or are MIA, missing in action.

Divers, Dogs, Despair, and Desolation

A few days after her disappearance, Chelsea's body turns up in a shallow grave covered with debris. Her body is only half a mile from where she parked her BMW. She was spotted by divers working the nearby lake. There is rage in the community. "Chelsea's blood on you, move out," someone spray paints in large red letters on the garage door of the suspect's mother.

Could this have all been so easily avoided by protecting the victims *before* the crime? Or could the horrifying truth be that we—as a society—*are addicted to the drama of violence?*

Junk Justice

The rage would be better directed at our broken justice system, which would be laughable if it weren't so utterly tragic. Why wasn't Chelsea warned about the previous attack on a female jogger in that same park? Why weren't there signs posted in that park? We post signs for falling rocks. We post warnings when a hungry coyote is spotted sniffing around for food. Why didn't anyone give this young woman the facts she needed to make *an informed judgment* about whether she wanted to go running in that park by herself when a sex predator was on the loose?

Why wasn't a suspect sketch obtained from Candice Moncayo, the December victim who got away? Cops reportedly lamented that Candice went back to Colorado. So? Couldn't the cops have hired a sketch artist in Colorado? Couldn't they have flown to Colorado to get the sketch? Couldn't cops have worked on a videoconference system, like Skype, to obtain the sketch? Here's the likely rationalization: *What's the big deal? Candice is okay. She didn't get hurt. It's not a priority. Besides, we don't have the budget.*

Our Justice System Is Reactive, Not Proactive

This case is typical. Let me pause to say that my observations are not directed at the rank-and-file men and women in blue who patrol our streets. I admire the police. Cops are overwhelmingly decent, hard-working, brave men and women who put their lives on the line for strangers on a daily basis. As a reporter, I've worked with beat cops for years and am in awe of their resilience in the face of a daily onslaught of the worst human nature has to offer. I feel safer because there are cops on the street in my neighborhood. However, there is a huge blind spot in our criminal justice system. Law enforcement, as a cultural institution, is really not all that interested in prevention. Prevention is boring. Prevention is really dull, hard work that offers no drama. Prevention, while it stops crime from happening, sometime in the indeterminate future, is like a tasteless glass of water.

It's Hard to Claim Credit for Stopping a Crime That Never Happened

If prevention is like a tasteless glass of water, then hunting for suspects, detective work, and forensics is like a bottle of champagne. It sparkles. It fizzes as it goes down. Prevention doesn't give us the adrenaline rush every addict craves. Crime and punishment does. Our culture is addicted to the charge we get from the whodunit suspense of crime: *Who did it and what's his motive? How did he get away? Did anyone see him? What's the evidence? How do you catch him?* Chases, cornering the criminal, the trial, closing arguments, and the sentencing, it's all very dramatic and much more exciting than drab, dull prevention. If you don't believe me, try attending a murder trial and see if you don't get nervous and filled with anticipation as the jury files in to announce their verdict. The inherent drama of violent crime is what makes it such perfect material for TV shows. There are no crime dramas about the prevention of crime!

"If anything is going to take longer than a single electoral cycle it's very, very difficult to get policy makers to buy into it. Unless there is some visible, tangible outcome that they can point to and say 'I did this' or 'I was behind this particular piece of legislation that had this outcome,' with a two- or four- or six-year cycle, it's tough for them to see it as in their best self-interest to back it."

—*Travis Pratt, author of* Addicted to Incarceration: Corrections Policy and the Politics of Misinformation in the United States

We, as a culture, much prefer to pull out all the stops, dive into action, and leave no stone unturned *after* the rape and murder. The politically incorrect, unspoken truth is this: the horror of a violent crime is like a line of cocaine that gives us a buzz, energizes us, and propels us into action. Our justice system prefers to spend untold millions of tax dollars sealing off the crime scene, searching for a victim, dusting for fingerprints, testing DNA, offering rewards for information, issuing all-points bulletins, arresting the suspect, holding news conferences, arranging a "perp walk" of the defendant so the media can get a close-up visual of him on camera, gathering evidence, formally charging him, setting the bail, holding the preliminary hearing, fighting over pretrial motions, selecting the jury, preparing witness lists, delivering opening arguments, cross-examining witnesses and experts, presenting closing statements, reading the verdict, hiring psychiatrists to assess the defendant, listening to the impact statements of the victims in the sentencing phase of the trial, and then locking up, feeding, clothing, and guarding the killer . . . rather than spend a tiny sliver of that cost preventing his crime in the first place. This addictive mind-set is a crime in itself.

Like so many others before him, John Gardner had a disturbing rap sheet. Ten years earlier, this same character had lured a thirteen-year-old girl home on the pretext of watching *Patch Adams,* a movie starring Robin Williams. Once he got the girl home, he attacked her. The DA's sentencing document says Gardner began "Rubbing his erect self against her private parts . . . got on top of victim . . . put his hand down the victim's pants . . . hit victim repeatedly in the face while rubbing himself and touching the victim in her private area under her clothes and sucking her breast over her clothes." The girl was begging for him to stop while crying. She says she felt like she was suffocating. She says she thought she was going to be raped. Eventually, she managed to run out the door "with only one shoe on, holding her pants" because they were unzipped. As a result of the pummeling Gardner gave her, the thirteen-year-old suffered a "laceration to the inside of her lip, a contusion under her left eye, bruising around the left eyelid area, numerous bruises on the left side of her head and face" plus other injuries.

John Gardner reached a plea deal in that attack and was sentenced to six years in prison. He got out after five years. Five years for molesting and pummeling a child! If he had been prosecuted to the full extent of the law, he might have gotten thirty years. Had the girl been raped and murdered, he might have even gotten the death penalty. But, hey, like Candice would a decade later, this thirteen-year-old got away before he could carry out the actual rape. So, even though the prosecutor's own report describes Gardner as extremely predatory and without "one scintilla of remorse," he gets a six-year sentence and is out in five.[1] Wow!

In the prosecution's 2000 sentencing report, a psychiatrist warns that John Gardner will attack girls again. A year earlier, he had fondled a fourteen-year-old girl's breasts and vaginal area and was never prosecuted at all. The activity was considered consensual, as if a fourteen-year-old has the capacity to give an informed consent to anything sexual.[2]

A few days after Chelsea's body was found, fourteen-year-old Amber DuBois's body was discovered by authorities. Amber had disappeared on her way to school less than eight miles from where Chelsea King vanished. Gardner was immediately described as the focus of the investigation into that girl's murder as well. Amber's case had gone unsolved for a year when Chelsea's murder, nearby, suddenly reactivated interest in what had become a cold case. Amber's mom revealed to me live on *Issues* that, when Amber first disappeared, cops waited three crucial weeks before pulling out all the stops to search for her daughter.[3]

Ultimately, John Gardner confessed to sexually assaulting and murdering both Amber DuBois and Chelsea King and was sentenced to life in prison without the possibility of parole. The families of both victims expressed anger and disappointment in how the criminal justice system handled John Gardner.[4]

America's Crime Machine Functions on Autopilot

After Chelsea's body was discovered, the community came together in an emotionally charged candlelight memorial several thousand strong. Again, the rites of America's addiction to violence have become all too predictable. We're all swept up in the drama, including me. I am certainly not suggesting that memorials not be held. It was obviously a tremendous comfort to the grief-stricken King family, who have shown enormous grace and vowed to devote their lives to preventing another needless death. But I'll bet my condo on this: the King family would gladly forsake that huge memorial if they could only have their daughter back.

The time for action is *before* the next horrific killing. We need to take all the energy we apply *after* the fact, including vigils and memorials, and harness that people-power to change this bankrupt system and prevent future senseless killings. But that won't give us the quick fix that we, an *Addict Nation*, crave.

Defining Crime Addiction

Addiction is an overpowering compulsion to use a substance or exhibit a behavior repeatedly despite consistently dire consequences. The pattern of addiction is an endless cycle of craving, bingeing (sometimes followed by remorse), and withdrawal, which sparks a new craving.

This perfectly describes America's approach to crime. Let's look at it for what it is. We all find sensational murder cases fascinating, myself included. Year after year, TV ratings have consistently shown that high-profile murder cases are guaranteed ratings grabbers. We *binge* on the coverage and almost simultaneously experience *remorse*. These stories are so gruesome, we tell ourselves, "They're hard to watch," even as we remain glued to the coverage. These horrific crimes make almost everything else—politics, the environment, education, international affairs—seem dishwater-dull by comparison.

If America goes too long without a sensational case, we experience *withdrawal*. A *craving* arises for another huge story. We're jonesing for another fix. Soon, we hit upon the next monstrous case and begin soaking up all the gory, new details.

Our Nation's Addiction to Crime Dictates How a Murder Case Itself Is Handled

A horrible, violent crime occurs. Neighbors feel a charge as they express outrage. Police feel the adrenaline rush of a high-profile case. They're pumped up to hit the streets and question potential witnesses. They display a competitive zeal to crack the case. Every resource is poured into solving it. Just as an alcoholic doesn't think of his family budget when he goes on a drinking spree, when crime reaches the crisis point of a sensational murder, then budgets be damned, money is no object!

The *binge* of effort soon gives way to a collective sense of *remorse* and sadness over the crime, which takes the form of vigils, memorials, funerals, and the creation of foundations and laws in the name of the victim: Jessica's Law and Megan's Law being just two examples. Thanks to these well-meaning efforts, a solution seems at hand. Hope returns. Until the next horrific murder when the pattern starts all over again.

We Are All Unconsciously Under the Sway of This Addictive Pattern

Let me stress that none of this is malicious or intentional. Everybody, including myself, feels obligated to carry out our assigned roles in this addictive drama. Most everyone, from law enforcement to the media, means well. But that's the nature of addiction. Cravings are baffling, powerful, and cunning. Addictions overwhelm our intellect and take it hostage. In the throes of our addiction, we "forget" the reasons we should be sober and reach for our vice by reflex—despite the wreckage we create in the process. So, we find ourselves justifying irrational, self-destructive cycles of crime glorification because we've lost control. The addiction rules us and turns us into mindless zombies on a constant mission to get the fix. We have become so powerless over the process that we now accept and expect that there will always be more and more horrific crime to report about in the United States. In fact, when something good happens, we rarely notice. It's hard to make headlines unless at least a few people are hurt in the process.

However innocent our intentions, we must face the truth, namely that this play is a tragedy of Shakespearean proportions that consistently ends in heartbreak and shattered lives. America needs a script doctor who will rework the story line, getting rid of our fascination with pain and violence and replacing it with evolved, sober, rational, proactive, preventative, compassionate approaches to our crime problem.

"When you look at our society, which is so heavily saturated in violence, there is an opportunity and an opening here for us to begin to explore the potential of creating structure within our society that would help us as individuals, families, and groups lead more peaceful lives. Once people start shooting, it's a little bit late to start talking about programs to create peace."

–*Dennis Kucinich, Congressman (D-OH)*

When an addict finally tires of the vicious cycle of addiction and decides to seek help, it's called "hitting bottom." America needs to hit bottom on our crime habit.

Addiction is as old as humankind. In all of history, there has only been one effective antidote to addictive behavior. It's called the Twelve Steps of recovery. These Twelve Steps, a distillation of timeless spiritual principles, came into the national consciousness through Alcoholics Anonymous, which was founded in the late

1930s and has since grown into a global force with millions of members.[5] The Twelve Steps operate on the premise that addiction is a form of "spiritual bankruptcy."

As it stands, our criminal justice system is cynical, jaded, lazy, complacent, and often corrupt. In terms of justice, it is spiritually bankrupt. Think I'm exaggerating? Well, let's look at how lazy, complacent, and jaded "the system" was in the case of John Gardner. Not only did they sentence him to five short years in jail for beating and molesting a thirteen-year-old girl, but—once he was out on parole—he brazenly defied the terms of his parole at least a half a dozen times and was not punished! Records show parole officials caught Gardner illegally living near a school. Yet they stamped his paperwork "COP," Continue on Parole, despite this offense. Parole officials acknowledge that Gardner also repeatedly let the battery on his GPS tracking device run low. He also missed a meeting with his parole officer. And each time Gardner thumbed his nose at the rules, he got the same response from our lazy, cynical system: COP, continue on parole, COP, COP, COP, COP, COP! Can you say COP OUT?

When asked about the failure to revoke Gardner's parole for repeated violations, a corrections official said, "These are considered minor. Quite frankly, if we were to blanket the system of parolees with minor offenses, we would . . . overwhelm the system." WHAT? So essentially the corrections department is admitting that parole rules are a joke and criminals can violate the terms of parole with impunity without fear of consequences. Does this seem outrageous? The idea that the system is incapable of enforcing its own rules with regard to violent sexual offenders is mind-boggling and the potential repercussions are grave—literally. This man was free to hurt and kill other women and girls while nearby prisons burst at the seams with nonviolent inmates doing time for drug offenses. After all, those offenses are a slam dunk to prosecute. You catch someone with drugs and it's game, set, match.

Just days after his last violation, Gardner was let off parole and his GPS tracking device was taken off his ankle. He was now totally free! That was in the fall of 2008. A few months later, Amber DuBois vanished while walking to school. The next year, Chelsea King was also dead.

The parole official justifies his department's lackadaisical attitude this way, "There was nothing to indicate that he would ... do this ... I guess one can always look back, but we don't have that luxury." We don't have the luxury to enforce the rules? Are you kidding me?

Oh, but I guess we had the "luxury" of letting Candice Moncayo get tackled and assaulted on a jog. I suppose we had the "luxury" of letting Chelsea King and Amber DuBois get sexually assaulted and murdered? Outrageous!

There was plenty to indicate Gardner was likely to attack again. A decade earlier, a psychiatrist warned he would! Do you see now how our system acts like the junkie who nods off and forgets to pay his bills or even bathe but is suddenly propelled into action when his body demands the next fix?

"If a criminal justice agency were to pursue this offender early on, in the hopes that the benefit would come later—five, ten, fifteen years down the road in terms of incapacitation—that's more difficult for them to get behind because they can't claim credit for that benefit. What they can do is, when something horrific happens, immediately jump into action. They can demonstrate the benefit—'Look how many people we're putting on this particular case. Look at the resources we're devoting to this. Look at how hard we're working.' The benefits become immediate. This is very consistent with the addiction metaphor. We don't do delayed gratification very well."

—Travis Pratt, associate professor at the School of Criminology and Criminal Justice, Arizona State University

Addiction to Crime Leads to Short-Term Thinking

Another excellent example of our "criminal justice junkie" mentality can be seen in the Jaycee Dugard case. Jaycee was eleven years old when she was abducted near a school bus stop. She was held for eighteen long years in a wretched warren of flimsy tents in a registered sex offender's backyard. Cops say Phillip Garrido raped Jaycee repeatedly and fathered two children by her who are now teenagers.

In 1976, more than three decades before Jaycee's case made national headlines, this same Phillip Garrido abducted Katie Callaway Hall after asking for a ride, on the pretext that his car was broken. He bound her and took her to a warehouse where, for seven long hours, he raped and tortured her. He was convicted and sentenced to half a century in prison. But they let this sex predator out after just over a decade. The system never even had the decency to inform Katie that the rapist, who made her existence a living hell, shattering her ability to trust others for years, was being released back into society early. Once out, Katie says Garrido proceeded to show up at her workplace, terrifying her again. Cops say it didn't take him long to resort back to his crime of choice: abduction and rape.

Phillip Garrido was on lifetime parole. He set up a home with his wife, Nancy, in California and was regularly visited by parole officers. Year after year, parole officers visited Garrido and never figured out that he was hiding three females captive in the ramshackle collection of tents in his backyard! Can you imagine that? Jaycee's two daughters grew up in that filthy hellhole, unable to even go to the doctor!

When they were teens, they were actually allowed to go to a neighbor's house for a party. So the neighbors were vaguely aware the Garrido kids existed but had no clue as to their hideous backstory. Then, in 2006, one neighbor finally sensed there was something horribly wrong at the Garrido household. That good citizen called 911 complaining that Garrido was psychotic and was keeping kids in his backyard. The caller swore the kids could be heard talking. So a cop visited Garrido, interviewing him on his front lawn. The officer concluded there was no evidence of criminality. That officer did not go into the backyard to check out the complaint for himself. That officer apparently did not know Garrido was a registered sex offender because he didn't check. Again, the broken ideals in our justice system are manifested in laziness, complacency, cynicism, and short-term thinking.

Phillip Garrido felt so invincible that he virtually had to shove his hostages in the face of the cops before they caught on. Phillip was only caught after he decided to take Jaycee and their two children (who thought Jaycee was their sister, not their mother) to a local university where he was preaching some bizarre philosophy related to his corporation/church called God's Desire. Finally, a couple of female campus cops noticed something suspicious. "He had two little girls with him and they didn't look right," said officer Lisa Campbell. Operating on what one of the officers called police intuition merged with mother's intuition, the female officers actually did some research and found out that Garrido was a sex offender on parole for kidnapping and rape. Then they called his parole officer.[6] The parole officer expressed surprise, insisting Phillip Garrido didn't have any children. Perhaps the female officers were mistaken? It gets worse.

Addicts Try to Cover Their Tracks

Addicts vehemently deny their responsibility even in the face of overwhelming evidence. After the scandalous story broke, and Jaycee and her teen daughters were reunited with Jaycee's traumatized mother, the California Department of Corrections and Rehabilitation tried to keep documents sealed that would show just how much they screwed up during their visits to Phillip Garrido's home for well over a decade![7]

The capper came many months later, long after the case made national news. California authorities were finally forced to admit that "agents saw and spoke to" Jaycee Dugard and her eldest daughter "but failed to investigate their identities or their relationship to Garrido." Yep! That's right! Parole agents actually spoke to the hostages, but were too clueless to even realize they were hostages and too lazy to do a little checking to find out who these young females hanging around with a convicted rapist/sex offender actually were. The state of California ultimately settled with Jaycee and her daughters, awarding the traumatized females $20 million.[8] So we pay people off after their lives are shattered but refuse to spend a fraction of that amount to prevent such crimes from happening.

If that true story does not prove our system's laziness, complacency, cynicism, and incompetence—in other words, spiritual bankruptcy—I don't know what does! Of course, once Jaycee was discovered, cops pulled out all the stops, as usual, pouring over every nook and cranny of Garrido's grotesque compound, collecting all sorts of vile evidence as they dismantled the backyard tents, charging Phillip and his wife with dozens of counts and pounding their chests over how they would send this sicko away! The system had him in the last century and they let him go! The addictive pattern of frantically cleaning up our messes only *after* the damage has been done is crystal clear. And it's obscene and destroying innocent lives.

Addiction Creates Fear and Paranoia; Sobriety Creates Serenity and Trust

These random stranger abductions of females are robbing virtually everyone in America of their peace of mind. Parents are terrified to let their children walk to the school bus alone . . . and with good reason. Adult women are forced into a psychological burka—fearful of going out alone to do an errand, drive to work, walk to the car in a parking lot, or even walk the dog.

If we developed a "sober" criminal justice system, we could eventually achieve peace of mind for all Americans. In place of the horror and drama of rape and murder, we could have prison sentences that mean what they say and parole officers who do more than go through the motions for parole violations. But that would mean reordering our collective priorities to put prevention first. As we've just outlined, right now prevention is considered a "luxury" we can't afford and put at the bottom of the criminal justice totem pole. It's this short-term, quick-fix thinking that is literally killing us!

Criminal as Addict

We have just looked at our cultural addiction to the drama of crime and violence from the "macro" perspective, where the masses are swept up into a collective ritual that results in our social systems falling into disastrously destructive patterns. But addiction to violence is also apparent in its "micro" manifestations, namely individuals who are hooked on the rush of committing crime—perpetrators who get high on violence and mayhem.

"As a street youth who engaged in a lot of criminal activity in the housing projects in Detroit, one of the primary goals was to have that feeling of empowerment because you felt that you had power over people. And people are addicted to power."

—Judge Mathis, district court judge and
syndicated television show judge

News reports describe the monster who murdered Amber DuBois and Chelsea King as a "convicted sex offender" and a "sexual predator." Those are labels that don't fully explain his behavior. To me it seems pretty obvious that John Gardner is, first and foremost, a "violence addict." It would appear that, in Gardner's psyche, violence has become enmeshed with sex, and sex has become intertwined with violence. So, in Gardner's sick mind, a state of sexual arousal might lead to thoughts of committing violence against a young female. And fantasies about hitting a girl would similarly lead him to become aroused sexually.

Intertwined compulsions are common. A lot of alcoholics smoke heavily when they drink, sometimes crystal meth addicts report developing an addiction to porn, and marijuana users are notorious for having a preoccupation with food known as the "munchies." Cross-addiction is where one addictive substance provokes a craving for another. Vodka and Valium is apparently such a popular combination for addicts that they even have a nickname for it: V and V.

Since all addiction is progressive, it's completely predictable that the behavior of criminals will escalate into ever more serious crimes. Again, a hallmark of addiction is when the addict needs more and more of the same substance or activity to achieve the same level of intoxication because he/she develops a tolerance for the drug of choice. Gardner beat and fondled a thirteen-year-old girl in 2000. A decade later, he was charged with rape and murder.

In 1999, a year before John Gardner attacked the thirteen-year-old in San Diego, a medical criminologist in England was telling the British Science Association that criminals can get hooked on the "buzz" of committing crime. "Some criminal activity may be best understood by a kind of addictive process . . . they get more tied up with the excitement, stimulation, and the buzz of committing the crime itself," said John Hodge, head of professional practice at one of England's largest high-security psychiatric hospitals.[9] Essentially, he's saying that criminals can get intoxicated or "high" on breaking the law. He urged rehabilitation to take into account the addictive nature of crime. While John Gardner was certainly not a good candidate for rehabilitation, there are plenty of other criminals who might be. Just as there are Twelve Step programs for treating alcoholics and drug addicts, there should be a Twelve Step program for treating violence addicts. If we stop the addictive cycle of crime in the earliest possible stage, we could progress toward preventing physical violence altogether.

An Act of Violence Is an Addictive Binge

In recovery we say that the one thing addicts cannot afford is resentment. Resentments build as we replay encounters and experiences that make us angry over and over again in our minds. The process of resentment can, in fact, be it's own form of mental addiction as we get a perverse pleasure from repeatedly reexperiencing our anguish. The tragic dichotomy is that many criminals lash out precisely because they have a victim mentality as a result of the resentments boiling up inside of them. They feel wronged and want somebody to pay, even if it's a total stranger. After his arrest, John Gardner gave a jailhouse interview where he complained his life was filled with mistreatment and disappointment. He explained his crimes by saying an uncontrollable rage burst from him and he could not stop attacking the two teenage girls he killed.[10] Resentment is more likely to trigger an addictive binge than any other emotion. It is an addicted state of mind.

Codependent on Crime

While criminals can get their "buzz" from committing a crime, most law-abiding Americans get their buzz from *watching others* commit crimes. We're the voyeurs of violence. I admit I used to love watching true-crime shows. I would curl up in a blanket and watch episode after episode, telling myself that I was learning all about the intricacies of evidence collection. But, truth be told, I was getting a certain rush from watching somebody else's life implode in violence. That's hard for me to admit, but it's true. The world is a scary place, and the cosmos is totally terrifying. Misfortune can spring up out of nowhere. Sinister forces lurk in dark corners waiting to pounce. But I was observing it all from the safe and snug confines of my living-room couch! The danger I was seeing unfold on the screen made me feel lucky and safe by comparison. I looked forward to each new episode. I was being codependent on crime and criminals.

Codependency Is Basically Addiction One Step Removed

The codependent is the person who is "hooked" on the addict. They are psychologically and emotionally captivated by the drama surrounding the drug or alcohol user. Their drug of choice is the person. The alcoholic husband, who is always going on benders and getting into jams, often has a "sober" wife who is unconsciously drawn to the excitement of living with the out-of-control alcoholic. "What is going to happen next?" she frets. She alternately scolds him and covers for him. Secretly, she may feel her life is more exciting because of the caretaker role she's taken on, which she internally dramatizes into a mission of heroic proportions. She is the voyeur getting off on the commotion of his addiction. On a deeper level, she may be reworking the trauma of a childhood incident: abandonment, rejection, or a disconnected family.

We need to ask ourselves, "What is at the core of the excitement we feel watching crime unfold on our TV sets or in the movies?" What does it do for us to go to the theater and plunk down fifteen bucks in order to watch a maniacal murderer terrorize a young woman? Do we "get off" on it? Do we temporarily forget our mundane problems because the violence on the giant screen is so compelling that it completely distracts us from everything else? When we see something horrible happen to someone else, either in the movies or in real life, do we feel safe and secure by comparison? When crime and violence are simply viewed as a curiosity, something to distract and entertain us, something to make us feel better about the disappointments in our lives, something that allows us to feel lucky by comparison, then we are using it as a way of self-medicating and escaping—as a drug.

When we buy a ticket for a front-row seat to the glamorized gore, then we, as the viewers and audience members, become the "users." We use violent crime for entertainment. We digest it as news. We consume a diet based on violence.

Watching Violence Propagates Violence

Consuming violence as entertainment conditions us to use violence to solve our problems, even when there are alternatives. A coyote in your backyard? Shoot it. Ask questions later. But, then, when horrific violence hits us directly—a murder, a home invasion, a violent kidnapping, or rape—we are still shocked. Why? When *we* have been luxuriating in the environment that spawns violence, when *we* have been subsidizing the promoters of violence!

Don't Buy Violence

2010 Sundance Film Festival. During a screening of the ultraviolent film *The Killer Inside Me,* a female audience member was so nauseated by the vicious beating the prostitute (played by Jessica Alba) gets from the sheriff (played by Casey Affleck) that she screamed out at the director, "How dare you?!" Good question. How did he dare to make a scene where Alba has her face so badly smashed that her jawbone is exposed, a movie so graphic that one professional reviewer admitted he bolted halfway through, unable to watch another frame of the film's explicit sadism. In the Q&A afterward, the director used the old *it's art* excuse, claiming, "It's not only just about what a killer is like or how a killer behaves. It's also kind of a very dramatic version of how we all are." I hate to say it, but he has a point. If we are all enjoying violence on some level and in some form, how can we point the finger at him? He's just taking our worst impulses to their logical extreme. Violence begets violence. The moment we partake in violence, we lose the moral high ground to object to somebody else's exploitation of it.

Basically, the director threw the issue back in our faces, saying, *Look in the mirror. What's your relationship with violence?*

Pretend Violence Is Real Violence

If you've ever watched a movie about serial killers and then lay paranoid in your dark bedroom hoping you've locked every window, or seen a kid run out of a movie theater yelling a mighty battle cry and throwing karate chops after seeing a film about war, you know that watching violent programming can make some people more fearful, while others become more aggressive. But can a movie that might simply scare the average viewer lead a mentally unstable person to commit a real assault or murder? We really cannot say that watching violence is harmless. Our life experience tells us it is not. Put another way, there is the possibility of a karmic kickback to watching violence. The subconscious mind can't be counted on to distinguish between pretend violence and real violence. We react physically to a scary movie by gasping or jumping in our seats because our psyche is processing the violence as if it were real. So, if we're indulging in violent movies, it's almost like we're subsidizing violence itself.

The Pushers

Violence is an easy fix for Hollywood. In order to cover their enormous production costs, producers need to make movies that appeal to a world market. Violent movies are the genre of choice because they're easily translated and crosscultural. After all, brutality requires no subtitles. In fact, the more violent the movie, the easier it is to repackage to a global audience. Sadly, most of these types of movies are stamped "Made in the U.S.A."

Television is no better. Despite a decades-long national debate, the level of televised violence just keeps accelerating. An average American child will see 200,000 violent acts and 16,000 murders on TV by age eighteen. [11] The last two or three generations are the first in the history of humankind to be exposed to so many images of sadism and carnage.

A good way to end the insanity is to stop subsidizing the images of violence against us. We can say "enough" to movies and TV shows that equate masculinity with aggression and create a hunter-prey relationship between men and women.

If you don't believe women are victimized more than men—by men—in the movies and in everyday life, try this test: Ask a man if he would be afraid to go alone to a bar or camping or hitchhiking or hiking or walking at night. The answer is probably no. Women, on the other hand, would be considered foolish to do such a thing. They would be putting themselves in almost certain danger. The question then, is, *Why do we accept this violence against women?* Perhaps it is because we are desensitized to it by television and film, and unscrupulous filmmakers are counting on us to continue financing that process.

"Our surveys tell us that the more television people watch, the more they are likely to be afraid to go out on the street in their own community, especially at night. They are afraid of strangers and meeting other people. A hallmark of civilization, which is kindness to strangers, has been lost."

–*George Gerbner, author of* Reclaiming Our Cultural Mythology[12]

Choose What World You Want

Where does this all end? We currently tolerate the killing of about eight women each day in the United States.[13] Is that enough? The FBI says there are 89,000 rapes per year. And that's just those that are reported.[14]

If things continue to get worse, will women need escorts or buddies for everyday errands like grocery shopping, going to the mall, or getting the mail? Will professional wrestling and bloody "extreme fighting" overtake traditional sports like tennis, skiing, and baseball as the new national pastime? Will our society be completely monitored by surveillance cameras? Do we want a high-tech "dark ages"?

We Can Evolve Beyond Crime

Imagine a world without crime. There is no fear of being raped and murdered. Kids race through their neighborhoods with abandon, their parents secure in the knowledge that they are not going to end up in the car of a stranger with a sick obsession. It is safe to accept the help of a stranger. People stop locking their doors and stop stockpiling weapons. Money used to fight crime and treat the injured is freed up for discretionary spending by individuals who've seen their tax bills plummet.

Sounds crazy, doesn't it! It's a terrible comment on our state of affairs that even the suggestion of a peaceful and serene world sounds ridiculously naïve. If we lack the imagination to even envision a peaceful world, how the hell are we actually going to get there? Someone said to me, "Hey, in two thousand years there will probably still be murders, prisons, and prisoners." Perhaps, but we must aim for something better.

Question Crime Assumptions

Addiction is so overpowering that it leads to inertia. All available energy must be summoned to satisfy the insatiable craving, which leaves little energy for anything else. This is why the addictive mindset is so often fatalistic: *What will be, will be!* This is clearly seen in our addictive relationship with crime. The assumption is: evil is out there, and therefore tragedy is inevitable. This is how we rationalize our inaction. But the truth is that much of the horrible tragedy I report on night after night is completely preventable and avoidable.

Just as the alcoholic irrationally fears life without booze will be a mind-numbingly dull affair, so the crime addict subconsciously rationalizes that brutality is inevitable because he fears that life would be drab without the drama of violence, whether in real life or on the screen. After all, that would leave us watching "chick flicks" —a genre so named because of its themes around love, affection, and romance. But if we kicked the crime habit, we would see that— just as the newly sober alcoholic finds new interests and challenges—we, too, would find healthy substitutes for violence.

We need to bring matriarchal values to our national debate on crime, teaching nonviolence and conflict resolution in schools and developing early interventions and therapeutic techniques that break the cycle of violence from being handed down to the next generation. And, when someone does cross the line into assault on an innocent woman or child, they need to remain behind bars as long as there's any hint that they're capable of striking again. If they do ever get out, they need to be rigorously tracked with lifetime GPS.

What is the opposite of violence? It's peace. If we are to evolve beyond violence, we must completely overhaul our government institutions to direct them toward peaceful alternatives, like prevention and genuine rehabilitation. And you and I must practice peace ourselves, in every choice we make.

The famous serenity prayer says: *Grant me the serenity to accept the things I cannot change, the courage to change the things I can, and the wisdom to know the difference.* I do not serenely accept that crime in the United States must remain the way it is now because I really believe we can change it. Now we just need the courage to change.

Chapter Seven
THE PUNISHERS: Addicted to Incarceration

S itting in prison, right now as you read this, is a man in his late twenties who will be behind bars until his forties. He didn't kill anybody. He didn't injure anyone. His story is typical. DeJarion was born and raised in Texas. Except for one incident of youthful theft, he stayed out of trouble. He graduated from high school with high hopes. As a star athlete, he was thrilled to find out he made a college football team, but then learned they didn't offer full athletic scholarships. Desperate for money to get into school and unable to find a job, DeJarion decided to make some quick cash by selling crack.

He had been selling crack for less than six months when his name surfaced as a drug dealer and his home was raided. Cops found 44 grams of crack cocaine and an unloaded rifle under his bed, along with about six thousand dollars in cash. At the age of twenty-three, DeJarion was sentenced to twenty years in prison. He will be a middle-aged man before he sees the outside of a jail cell again.

At the sentencing, the judge himself seemed revolted at the penalty he was legally required to impose because of mandatory drug-sentencing laws, lamenting, "This is one of those situations where I'd like to see a Congressman sitting before me." DeJarion left behind a fiancé and two young daughters, who will be all grown up before their daddy finishes living out the prime of his life in a cage. DeJarion is African-American and low income.[1] Fair? Well, let's see.

Lindsay Lohan was arrested in 2007. After an argument at a party in Malibu, witnesses claim the troubled movie star commandeered someone else's SUV. A young man claimed to TMZ that Lindsay ran over his foot with the vehicle before going on a high-speed chase down the Pacific Coast Highway.[2] Two other young men complained on camera to the website that they just happened to be sitting inside the SUV when the starlet jumped into the driver's seat and raced off. They say they found themselves terrified but unable to stop Lindsay. They claim she reached speeds of 100 miles an hour while boasting, "I can't get in trouble. I'm a celebrity. I can do whatever the fuck I want."[3] Turns out she was right! Lindsay allegedly chased after a woman who was so frightened she called 911 and drove straight to the Santa Monica police station, with Lindsay on her tail. When caught, cops say Lindsay had cocaine on her.

Lindsay already had a history of drunk driving. "What Miss Lohan did that night was extremely dangerous and reprehensible," said the woman who filed a lawsuit against Lohan over the incident. "Someone could easily have been killed or seriously hurt because of her irresponsible decisions that evening."[4] Despite all this, Lindsay Lohan was only charged with a handful of misdemeanors, including DUI and reckless driving, and got probation.[5] Might someone else less powerful have been charged with kidnapping, vehicular assault, or even carjacking? You betcha! Lindsay then proceeds to violate the terms of her probation and misses a crucial court date while off in France. Finally, she is sent to the slammer. She is released in less than two weeks. Lindsay, as we all know, is white, famous, and has made millions.

Then there's Cameron Douglas. The troubled son of movie star Michael Douglas was busted in a pricy Manhattan hotel for dealing drugs. Cops say Cameron played the middleman in a deal involving a half a pound of crystal meth. Initially, Cameron was allowed to remain under house arrest at his mother's multimillion-dollar Manhattan apartment while monitored by a private security company. Then, cops say, his girlfriend was caught trying to smuggle heroin past the guards to Cameron in an electric toothbrush.[6] Cameron had previous drug arrests and has had a serious drug problem since he was thirteen years old.[7]

Hoping to influence Cameron's sentencing, his famous father wrote an impassioned letter to the federal judge. So did actress Catherine Zeta-Jones, the suspect's superstar stepmother. Another letter came from the suspect's grandfather Kirk Douglas of *Spartacus* fame. Yet another missive came from legendary basketball coach Pat Riley. It was a campaign for leniency, carried out by heavy hitters, and it worked. Cameron was sentenced to just five years in prison when he could have gotten a decade. With time served and credit for in-prison programs, he could be out in three years.

As part of the deal, reports claim Cameron ratted out a couple of his drug suppliers, a pair of Latino brothers who were arrested on trafficking charges and could face life in prison.[8]

If you're noticing a certain disparity here, you're not imagining things. Hundreds of thousands of poor minorities are serving sadistically long terms in prison for low-level, nonviolent drug crimes. Whites are less likely to be arrested and much more likely to get either no prison time or a much shorter sentence. Our society evidently suffers from a bad case of selective indignation.

There are a few reasons for this. For decades, the laws on the books have been much harsher for crack cocaine, which is more likely to be used by blacks than powder cocaine, which is more likely to be used by affluent whites. In the summer of 2010, the Fair Sentencing Act was finally signed into law by President Obama.[9] It goes a long way toward closing the gap between sentences for crack versus sentences for powder cocaine. But it only applies to people convicted in federal courts. And, if you're already in the slammer, sorry, but it doesn't apply to you. Imagine how that feels.[10]

"One of the things that we know is that we over-police urban areas. When you put more police in an area, you naturally find more crime. We focus on a particular population and that population ends up incarcerated."

—Donna Selman, author of Punishment for Sale

One big reason a disproportionate number of low-income African-Americans are in prison is attitude. There is a culture of indifference in our criminal justice system toward Americans who are poor and powerless, and those individuals are primarily low-income blacks and Hispanics. In my thirty years as a reporter, I've seen the inconsistency play out again and again, and I would be willing to testify there's a cultural compulsion to incarcerate the underclass!

Don't get me wrong. Prisons have an important place . . . for murderers, rapists, armed robbers, child molesters, and the like. But today in America, we are locking up so many petty, nonviolent offenders that, ironically, we often have no room for the genuinely dangerous predator . . . who gets released from prison in order to relieve overcrowding.

As discussed earlier, John Gardner served only five years for admittedly beating and fondling a young girl. After his release, he repeatedly violated the terms of his parole but was still not arrested because—said a parole official—doing so would "overwhelm" the system due to prison overcrowding. Remaining free, John Gardner went on to sexually assault and murder two beautiful teenage girls in Southern California, Amber DuBois and Chelsea King. Meanwhile, minorities serving mandatory sentences for nonviolent crimes are doing twenty years for being caught with some crack under their bed.

Americans have lost perspective on punishment. We've become drunk on a "lock 'em up and throw away the key" cocktail, fixated on the satisfaction we feel when we hear a "tough sentence." Sadly, poor minorities are drowning in the wreckage of our addiction.

For years, when I was a reporter on the syndicated TV show *Celebrity Justice*, I would go to the Los Angeles criminal courthouse for a celebrity case and find myself sitting through a few non-celebrity cases as I waited for the star defendant to arrive. The difference between how the rich and the poor were treated in the very same courtroom was simply breathtaking.

For the poverty-stricken defendants, who are represented by public defenders, it seemed like the whole system was on speed. The prosecutor, the judge, and the public defender would banter—often cheerfully—using legalistic, acronym-filled language, without any real acknowledgment that a human being was sitting there with his life in the balance. I could hardly keep up. At the end of a flurry of chatter, the public defender would mumble a recommendation to the person on trial. The defendants often seemed confused. Their English was sometimes poor. The offer was usually some kind of plea deal, and the clueless defendant invariably agreed. Within seconds, he would be carted off to prison to be replaced by another poor, minority defendant. As one former prosecutor confided in me, "When I looked out at the cases on the docket, all I could see was a sea of black and brown faces." A poor person trapped in the criminal justice system is just a number, a commodity to be sorted and stocked.

By contrast, I noticed with dismay, when the rich and famous defendant arrived, often with a team of high-powered attorneys, the judicial process would begin to move in slow motion. The judge, prosecutor, and the defendant's dream team of attorneys would interminably dissect every last nuance of every legal maneuver. There were frequent huddles at the judge's bench, out of earshot of the journalists on hand. Often, the entire proceeding would end up being postponed due to some well-presented excuse and we, reporters, were left to come back another day. No, justice isn't blind. In fact, Lady Justice seems to have undergone LASIK surgery. Now, she's just terribly short-sighted.

Most imprisoned Americans are poor, male, and members of a minority group. Roughly two-thirds of the United States population is white. But white males comprised only about one-third of the inmate population in 2007. Hispanics, who can be of any race, are about 15 percent of the American population, but Hispanic males accounted for about 18 percent of all inmates. African-Americans comprise only about 13 percent of the population. But black males represented the largest percentage—35 percent—of all inmates held in custody in 2007.[11] In other words, more than half of all inmates are minority, way above their percentage in the general population. The question is "Why?"

Is there something wrong with minorities? How ridiculous. That would be a highly racist concept. And you certainly wouldn't hear that from me, since I am a woman of color, being Puerto Rican on my mother's side. Do I need to remind anyone that we have an African-American president? Even those who might disagree with some of his policies would never mistake him for a dummy! Ditto for Puerto Rican Supreme Court Justice Sonia Sotomayor! Nevertheless, if you toured the nation's prisons and looked at the racial makeup, you might wonder . . . why are so many people of color locked up? America's prison system today is a case study in institutionalized racism. And it's hurting all of us . . . black, brown, and white. We're relying almost entirely on one solution—incarceration—to deal with myriad complex social problems. It's simplistic, and it's morally wrong. But we're culturally hooked on doing it this way.

"We have an addiction to a false sense of justice. Punishment is the mentality rather than rehabilitation."

—Matthew Albracht, managing director of the Peace Alliance

More Than 2 Million Americans Warehoused

Right now, as you read this, more than 2 million human beings are living in cages in America. That's about the same as the entire population of Slovenia . . . or Macedonia . . . or any number of countries.[12] In fact, America has more human beings locked up in prisons than any other country in the world. Here's another way to look at it: about one out of every 100 adults in the United States is in prison![13] More than 7 million Americans are either behind bars, on probation, or on parole.[14] We have 5 percent of the world's population but 25 percent of the world's prison population. Any which way you slice it . . . it's shocking! As a country, we are on a punishment binge, and when you consider that most addictive behavior is progressive, this trend is almost guaranteed to grow. So, it's high time we ponder the question: Why are we, as Americans, so obsessed with putting people behind bars?

Helter Skelter

The roots of America's fanatical need to incarcerate began back in the late sixties and seventies when our nation's crime problem seemed to be spinning out of control. August 9, 1969, is a date that will live in infamy throughout the hills of Southern California and the world. It was the night the Manson clan committed its savage massacre of Sharon Tate, the very pregnant wife of film director Roman Polanski, and four other people, including an heiress to the Folgers coffee fortune. Before leaving, the "family" scrawled the word "pig" in blood on the front door. In another viciously sadistic Manson clan slaying, the very next night the Beatles-inspired phrase "Healter-Skelter" was written and, yes, misspelled, in blood at that crime scene. The late author and social observer Dominick Dunne wrote, "The shock waves that went through the town were beyond anything I had ever seen before. People were convinced that the rich and famous of the community were in peril. Children were sent out of town. Guards were hired."[15] The killings also dealt an ultimately fatal injury to America's counterculture movement. Even though their philosophy was based on racism and violence, the Manson family looked like flower children. That was enough.

Average Americans, already feeling destabilized and threatened by the long-haired hippies who seemed to be everywhere, declared war on the peaceniks and their favorite pastimes, free love and mind-altering drugs. The author Joan Didion wrote, "Many people I know in Los Angeles believe that the sixties ended abruptly on August 9, 1969, ended at the exact moment when word of the murders on Cielo Drive traveled like brushfire through the community, and in a sense this is true. The tension broke that day. The paranoia was fulfilled."[16]

And from the ashes of those horrific killings would rise an anti-crime crusade that would ultimately end up imprisoning hundreds of thousands of young men who weren't even alive when Charlie Manson ordered his followers to murder.

Over the next few decades, the anticrime movement would create its own set of problems, taking down millions of uneducated young men and women, from the underclass, who were not violent but had broken the law. The consequences to families and communities have rippled across generations.

"Moms actually give birth in jail now, and the kids grow up visiting their mom in prison. You're seeing people who are going through their childhood with an incarcerated parent. There are these big, giant institutions that you are fighting to keep out of, but it kind of has this tractor beam attached. We heard the same story over, and over, and over, and over."

–Simeon Soffer, director of prison documentary film Fight to the Max

---

In the eye-opening book *Addicted to Incarceration*, author Travis Pratt writes, "One out of every three African-American men in the United States population between the ages of 20 and 29 is under some form of correctional supervision (prison, jail, probation, or parole); when limited to urban areas, that figure approaches 1 in 2 . . . a high rate of incarceration may indirectly increase crime rates through its effect on both family disruption and the potential economic deprivation brought on by the loss of an additional (or perhaps the only) income."[17] In the vicious cycle of our "lock 'em up" addiction, we destroy families by imprisoning parents and then watch the unsupervised, undisciplined children grow up to become criminals themselves. Our incarceration of minorities is a self-perpetuating, destructive process. And we justify it all with the word . . . *justice.*

Charlie Manson had hoped to provoke a war against blacks, which he called Helter Skelter. In a sick irony, he may have instigated just that.

Here Is the Backstory on
Our Addiction to Imprisonment

As the sixties gave way to the seventies and the eighties, a relentless crime wave swept across the nation. The violence seemed to rob Americans of a fundamental sense of security. A lot of the crime was random and horrific. Son of Sam came to epitomize the era. This mystery serial killer singlehandedly terrorized New York City from July 1976 until his arrest in August 1977. The phantom, who would turn out to be nerdy David Berkowitz, seemed to come out of nowhere and gun down strangers at random, particularly women with long, dark hair and couples parked in cars.[18] I was a college student living in New York City at the time and, as a young woman with long, dark hair, I was terrified, biting my lip anxiously as I walked around town, always looking over my shoulder for anybody who looked "strange."

The "establishment" became increasingly convinced that a hard line was called for. The pendulum started to swing from permissiveness to punishment. The notion spread that America was coddling criminals and needed to get tough. Politicians realized that campaigning for "law and order" increased their chances of getting elected. "Law and order" translated into tougher sentences. Conservatives chanted the mantra that rehabilitation is a joke. Victims of violent crime wanted vengeance, and who could blame them? It was said that a conservative is a liberal whose been mugged!

"The era of accelerated incarceration and punishment—being the primary purpose over deterrence and rehabilitation—began in the '70s when the law-and-order politicians and law-and-order candidates began to use the sensationalism of crime to scare voters into selecting them. If you ran for any office, for the most part, a principal part of your platform beginning in the

'70s had to be 'I will be tough on crime' not that 'I will reduce crime by changing lives and getting to the root causes.'"

–Judge Mathis, syndicated television show judge

Much of the violence was fueled by the burgeoning illegal drug trade. The middle class and the rich were creating a lot of the demand, doing drugs like crazy. But they could afford to snort a few paychecks up their noses. Low-income addicts often needed to rob—and sometimes kill—to pay for a habit that can get very pricey. The middle class and rich indulged in their "cool" habit behind gated walls and in penthouse apartments. The poor dealt and used their drugs right on the street. Coke was neatly laid out on a mirror, while crack vials littered the gutters. For these reasons, poor addicts and dealers were getting arrested in droves while middle- and upper-middle-class drug users—and their upscale drug suppliers— were not. I saw this myself as a young journalist in the 1980s. Looking back, I can say that it's a bizarre blessing that, as an alcoholic, my drug of choice was booze. I dabbled in drugs on a few occasions, but I consider myself lucky to have avoided picking up the habit I saw all around me. So many middle-class professionals were doing coke regularly that it was certainly not shocking to walk into a party full of yuppies and encounter a group in a corner, or in a quiet bedroom, doing lines. None of those people ever thought twice about being arrested because it so rarely happened to a hip, young, urban professional, no matter how strung out they got.

The fear of crime ultimately morphed into the so-called War on Drugs. This accelerated the disproportionate imprisonment of African-Americans, even though most drug users are white. While the tougher laws may have been designed—admirably—to cut down on violent crime, it became apparent that it was much easier to catch somebody with a stash of drugs than solve a complex murder case, a messy rape, or neighborhood robbery where everyone scatters. For example, nationally—in 2008—less than a third of all robberies were "solved" with an arrest. Less than half of all rapes were cleared with the capture of a suspect. But drug cases are often easy to prosecute. No DNA testing or complex forensics is required. No he said/she said to deal with. Just a hand on a stash and, for good measure, some cash!

In the 1980s, as First Lady Nancy Reagan urged Americans to "just say no," President Reagan ramped up the War on Drugs. The crime/drug nexus was fixed in the public's mind.

As we entered the 1990s, three-strikes laws began popping up in states across the nation, mandating long prison sentences for those convicted of a third felony. About two dozen states enacted three-strikes laws. All of this caused incarceration rates to explode. And who was taking the biggest hit? African-American males.

We, the Taxpayers, Are Paying for the Incarceration of So Many

Overcriminalization is a term now being used by both liberals, concerned about the exploitation of prisoners, and conservatives worried about big government. Liberals see the inequities in the arrest, conviction, and sentencing rates. Conservatives, whose entire philosophy is based on limiting the government's control over the lives of American citizens, are now looking with alarm at the escalating number of prisons and prisoners. The American Civil Liberties Union sums it up this way: "Between 1970 and 2005, the number of men, women, and children locked up in this country has grown by an historically unprecedented 700%."[19]

The Other "Pushers"

Just like drug cartels make billions off the drug trade, America's prisons have become big business, a business that has a vested interest in making sure that crime doesn't go away. Every time a prisoner phones home, somebody makes a profit. Inmate phone calls alone are a $1 billion market![20] There is now a prison/industrial complex where self-perpetuating prison bureaucracies have aligned with the private sector to create a massive industry based on locking people up. They even have their own magazine, *Corrections Today*, and a product-packed Las Vegas convention.

> "You walk in and it's absolutely every business from toothpaste suppliers that design special packaging for prisons, to telephone companies, the chairs, the restraints—every company that is feeding at this bulk of money that's been allotted for criminal justice and corrections [is] there. And it's lights and cameras, and the whole bit."
>
> —*Donna Selman, author of* Punishment for Sale

The American Correctional Association's yearly confab is like the auto show, except, instead of nifty new gizmos in cars, it showcases cool ways to house and control captive humans. Several hundred exhibitors show off their wares, everything from suicide-proof toilets to pre-fab prison cells. Here's a look at just one prison product in a $37 billion (and growing fast) prison industry.[21]

> "With 2-inch hollow steel walls, the cells feature built-in light-ing, beds, and plumbing. MaxWall, which typically sells for $14,000 to $18,000, is shipped like an erector set and stitch-welded together onsite. The cells can save 10 square feet of space each over conventional cell construction techniques, allowing prisons to accommodate more inmates."
>
> *—CNNMoney.com*

It costs more than $22,000 a year to feed and house the average prisoner. Some say it's actually a lot higher than that. But, for argument's sake, multiply that figure by the more than 2 million Americans who are locked up, and you get a taste of how much money is up for grabs.[22]

Lately, there has been a frightening trend toward privatizing prisons. This provides an even greater profit incentive to lock up as many people as possible. If you're in the prison industry, how do you "grow" your business? Imprison more Americans! Critics complain that the prison industry has a powerful lobby that pushes politicians to enact even tougher laws with even longer incarceration.

> "These are profit-driven, market-model industries, and their premise is to make money and increase market. Their market and, unfortunately, their raw materials are human beings."
>
> *—Donna Selman, author of* Punishment for Sale

"We feel very, very good about the business prospects," a Corrections Corporation of America (CCA) executive told *Business 2.0 Magazine.* The Nashville-based company is the largest private prison operator in the U.S., employing nearly 17,000 people and housing 75,000 prisoners. The company also has a subsidiary that transports prisoners. It reportedly racked up a profit of $47 million during the first six months of 2006 alone.[23] CCA is traded on the New York Stock Exchange under the ticker symbol CXW.[24] "Our core business touches so many things—security, medicine, education, food service, maintenance, technology—that it presents a unique opportunity for any number of vendors to do business with us," the executive added. On its website, CAA calls itself "the fifth-largest corrections system in the nation, behind only the federal government and three states."[25]

A Business . . . REALLY?

I think it's our responsibility to ask ourselves, *Is this something we really want to delegate to the private sector?* Do we, as American tax-payers, really want to underwrite a for-profit business that relies on humankind's darkest impulses to keep its doors open? It gives you that queasy feeling, doesn't it? But, wait, there's even more to keep you tossing and turning tonight as you think of the more than 2 million people in America who literally cannot get up and go to the kitchen to whip up a midnight snack! The Democratic Leadership Council estimates "about 100,000 of America's 2.3 million inmates of state, federal, and local prisons work in national and state prison industries."[26] That's right, I said they "work" in prison! The yearly sales total is around $2.4 billion." TWO BILLION DOLLARS!

And Now for Something Really Orwellian

Most Americans have no idea that something called UNICOR exists. That's the trade name for Federal Prison Industries, a wholly owned, government corporation that's been around since 1934 and was inspired by the Great Depression. It claims to keep inmates "constructively occupied" by getting them to churn out "market-priced quality goods and services for sale to the Federal Government" at more than a hundred prison factories. UNICOR/FPI claims to be "not about business, but instead, about inmate release preparation . . . helping offenders acquire the skills necessary to successfully make that transition from prison to law-abiding, contributing member of society."[27] The merchandise? "Merely by-products of those efforts." Hmmmm. By law, FPI must sell its products to the federal government. Its biggest customer is the Department of Defense, where it racks up more than half its sales.[28]

According to the *Left Business Observer*, the federal prison industry produces much of the U.S. military's helmets, ammunition belts, bulletproof vests, ID tags, shirts, pants, tents, bags, and canteens. But along with equipment for war, prison workers can also be found making paints, paintbrushes, appliances, headphones, and office furniture.[29] Many state prisoners hold jobs sorting public records—anything from tax files to student transcripts—for federal, state, and local governments. By the way, that means some convicts get to see Social Security numbers and other personal information about citizens on the outside—despite years of warnings that it's a dangerous practice.[30]

UNICOR's net sales in 2008 approached $1 billion. But . . . less than 5 percent of its revenue went to inmate pay. How's that possible? It's possible because UNICOR pays its captive workforce—of more than 20,000 prisoners—anywhere from twenty-three cents an hour to a top salary of $1.15 an hour.[31]

Critics call this slave labor. Some have even made the comparison to Nazi-era slave worker camps. Still others point out that prison labor also has its roots in slavery. After the Civil War, a system of "hiring out prisoners" was introduced in order to continue the slavery tradition.[32]

While I understand the argument for keeping prisoners occupied and productive, the irony becomes positively surreal when you consider that we are locking up armies of Americans for decades over nonviolent crimes and then telling them we are going to "help them" stay productive and "train them" for their re-entry to the real world by having them churn out goods (often on out-of-date, retired equipment) while earning a quarter per hour. Would that make you angry? You wonder why we often see these news stories of ex-cons engaged in horrific random violence against law-abiding citizens who've done nothing to deserve it. Well, a couple of decades behind bars provides a lot of time to build up rage, rage that is not directed at any single individual but rather at society as a whole.

The prison industrial complex fosters an us-versus-them mentality that can lead ex-cons to seek vengeance on the outside for humiliations endured on the inside. Sexual victimization by fellow inmates is a real problem that can scar an individual for life—leaving him bitterly resentful and ashamed. Prison overcrowding and punishment of inmates can create stress and rage. Ponder this one statistic: From 1995 to 2000, the number of offenders assigned to solitary confinement increased by 40 percent![33] Can you imagine what it feels like to be in solitary confinement? Can you imagine a guy being released onto the streets after a long period of severe isolation with no support system in place for him to transition back into society? How long do you think it will take for that man to get arrested again? And for what? Murder, robbery, rape?

In 1979, Congress allowed some private for-profit companies to hire prisoners in some limited circumstances if they're paid the prevailing wage.[34] Critics insist the wages prisoners get from private firms are, nevertheless, often substandard. Every so often a controversy will erupt where a big-name corporation is called out for using prison labor.[35] However, much more ominous than the occasional scandal is the relentless push by some politicians to legally throw the doors wide open to the widespread use of prison labor by private, for-profit corporations for egregiously substandard pay, literally pennies per hour. One critic put it best when he said that corporate America is salivating over the prospect of using more prison inmates for labor because businesses don't have to pay for a prisoner's health care, inmates belong to no union, they can't go on vacation, and they can't complain to the boss when they don't like the working conditions.[36] Are we, as a culture, at the doorstep of a new era of slavery, where it will be taken for granted that a large portion of the population is shackled, chained, and living in cages?

Despite all the talk of building skills in prison, we all have seen enough real crime stories to know the truth. Prisons are "criminal factories." A person who goes into prison comes out more of a hardened criminal than when he/she went in. They are marked for life and often have trouble getting hired because of their rap sheet. Recidivism is rampant. A few years ago, the Commission on Safety and Abuse in America's Prisons released *Confronting Confinement*, a scathing report on America's prison system. It noted, "Within three years, 67 percent of former prisoners will be rearrested," and most will be re-incarcerated.[37]

And the cost of it all? In 2006, the total tab just for prisons was $60 billion a year. And the bill is sure to have grown since then. That's your tax dollars. If it all sounds irrational, that's because addictive behavior is always ultimately irrational. We are drunk on crime and need an intervention to force us to look at some emotionally sober alternatives!

Imagine what we could do to change the culture that has led to so much imprisonment if we spent $60 billion on something positive ... like improving schools in inner-city neighborhoods that are pockets of crime. Imagine if we took $60 billion and put that into charter schools to replace public schools that are failing so miserably to educate America's underclass. Imagine if we put $60 billion into after-school programs that offer meaningful alternatives to gang membership. Imagine if we put $60 billion into family planning and birth control so that teenagers weren't giving birth with no viable means of supporting their infants. Imagine if we put $60 billion into psychological counseling programs so that kids from troubled or drug-ridden homes could have a place to vent and work out their emotional traumas.

"For every dollar we spend on substance abuse programs, we save seven in the long run, but we're not willing to make the front-end investment. You can take credit for catching a criminal, but you can't take credit for preventing a crime."

–*Donna Selman, author of* Punishment for Sale

Given that studies show the majority of inmates in American prisons have some kind of substance-abuse problem, imagine if we put $60 billion into treatment programs, rehabs, and halfway houses in the inner city.[38]

Imagine if we put $60 billion into vocational training so that young men in the inner city could learn a practical trade that would give them a shot at employability as a carpenter or an electrician ... so they wouldn't have to resort to drug dealing to survive. Europe offers students two options to gainful employment. For some, it's college and the professions. For others, it's learning a trade, like mechanics, plumbing, and electronics. The burgeoning solar industry needs technicians. The healthcare system needs skilled workers. But, today, vocational training is falling by the wayside in

America's high schools. Our education budgets are strained . . . while the budgets for prisons are skyrocketing.

The truth is a lot of undocumented workers cross the border from Mexico or Guatemala with much better practical skills than low-income Americans. Many undocumented workers know carpentry, how to lay cement, basic electrical work, how to lay hardwood floors, and so on. That's why Americans looking for cheap labor often hire illegals right in the parking lot of do-it-yourself superstores. Conversely, a lot of inner-city Americans grow up skillless! Wouldn't it be smarter to train young Americans before they end up in prison so they can get meaningful work instead of waiting for them to commit a crime out of financial desperation or hopelessness? Too often, they are incarcerated at huge public expense and, only there, trained inside prison for some theoretical future back on the outside. Wouldn't it be smarter to give tax breaks to corporations, large and small, to encourage them to become part of the solution by establishing partnerships and mentoring programs that fast track high-risk students into the workforce?

"I'm told it cost nearly $50,000 to house me in jail for those nine months. Six months later I got my GED and was admitted to college under an affirmative action program. My tuition, which included room, board, and classes, cost $6,000 per year. So I received a bachelor's degree on the back of taxpayers for $24,000—nearly half the amount it cost the taxpayers to keep me in jail for nine months. First of all, it was clearly more tax efficient to educate me than to incarcerate me because I was rehabilitated and didn't go through that revolving door, and secondly, I'm a pretty good taxpayer myself, helping to offset the pockets of others."

–Judge Mathis, district court judge and television show judge

---

Right now, in every city in America, there are poverty-stricken communities where a huge percentage of the population lives below the federal poverty line. In streets lined with abandoned buildings, young men—with no skills—languish, unable to get what they want or need through legal means. Many will automatically embark on a life of drugs and crime because they see absolutely no other alternative. They come from dysfunctional, broken homes where their adult role models are in and out of prison. They are functionally illiterate. Therefore, they cannot operate successfully in an increasingly complex society. At best, they can get dead-end, minimum-wage jobs. This is the core group that ends up in prison, generation after generation. But instead of working to break the vicious cycle of intergenerational criminality, we instead obsess about locking them up.

"We are so used to it and think that is the way to deal with things, and yet it doesn't work. The people that leave prisons get back on the streets and it's the same cycle. It's the cycle of violence, and if you don't break the cycle, you pay the costs one way or the other. And you pay it over and over and over again."

—Matthew Albracht, *managing director of the Peace Alliance*

As it stands today, many low-income, inner-city males are increasingly predestined to become a statistic in the criminal justice system. While America has recently become obsessed with making sure inner-city high schoolers know algebra, it would be wise to also fit in some classes on nonviolent conflict resolution. Why don't we create in-school programs to teach kids effective ways of dealing with their anger and shame? You might say, "Well, that's the job of the parent!" But, increasingly, in "the projects" the parent is in prison! According to the Bureau of Justice Statistics, in 2007, more than 1.5 million minor children had a parent in prison, more than 2 percent of all children in America. The City Mayor's Society adds, "Many more children have an incarcerated sibling or close relative. African-American children are much more likely to have an incarcerated parent. Seven percent of all black children in the United States have a parent who is currently incarcerated, compared with fewer than 1 percent of white children."[39] These children suffer shame, stigmatization, trauma, loneliness, and longing. At every moment in their young, formative years, they must live with an awareness that the person who brought them into this world is considered unworthy of being in public. How would that affect you psychologically? Would it hurt your self-esteem and make you depressed? The twenty-five-year-old daughter of a woman who was just nine years old when her mother was sentenced to decades in prison for conspiracy to distribute crack described the impact on her this way, "It made me numb. Things that made other people happy, I was nonchalant about."[40] That is one of the saddest things I've ever heard.

The Makings of a Moral Vacuum

When people feel worthless, when they feel they have absolutely nothing to lose, that's when they become really dangerous. How else to explain why incomprehensibly brutal acts of violence are so frequently in the news that they seem almost commonplace, even as the overall crime rate has decreased since the early 1990s?[41]

One particularly hideous story we covered on *Issues* continues to haunt me. It happened in one of the most crime-ridden public housing projects in Trenton, New Jersey. A seven-year-old girl went with her fifteen-year-old stepsister to a party in an apartment known for drug and gang activity. Cops say the older girl first prostituted herself with a group of men and then handed the child to them in exchange for more cash. Cops say the seven-year-old was gang-raped by a group of about five males ranging in age from their early teens to their twenties. One young suspect was only thirteen years old.[42] Now what could possess a thirteen-year-old boy to rape a seven-year-old girl? Peer pressure? It's a good guess that this boy grew up in an environment with virtually no moral guidance or loving discipline and under the influence of older males who had already become so morally corrupted they had morphed into sadists. That thirteen-year-old boy is also a victim . . . of emotional neglect and moral abandonment. Is locking him up for life really going to solve the problem in that housing project and others like it? Of course not! When we're churning out thirteen-year-old rapists, it should be an ear-piercing wake-up call to society that we need to intervene and do something besides "lock em up and throw away the key!"

Our Craving to "Punish"

The underlying problem? America's incarceration junkies regard drug programs, charter schools, vocational training, and family planning as a joke. They're boring (i.e., sober) alternatives. None of that is as potent as a hit of a good old-fashioned tough sentence. We want instant gratification—instant justice.

"Justice" has become an escape, and—yes—even a form of entertainment. Reality shows on cable TV are making money hand over fist telling stories from inside the walls of prisons, and we love to watch! We love seeing the humiliation of prisoners forced to squat for body cavity searches. Their dehumanization makes for good TV! Chain gangs are back! Society applauds the sheriff who insists on loud prison stripes or even makes male prisoners wear pink to demean them. We vicariously relish the revenge prison stabbing that's caught on surveillance tape because we feel so powerless against criminals in the outside world. It gives us a rush and a sense of control. We crave it again and again. We are incarceration junkies.

From Punishment to Prevention

So where will it end? When half the population is imprisoned and the other half lives behind fortress walls cowering in fear? When we try eight-year-olds as adults, locking them up for life? Is that the kind of future we want? Let's have a moment of clarity! Let's admit that we are intoxicated with the notion of punishment and need to open our minds and our hearts to emotionally sober alternatives that will prevent people from developing into criminals.

It is possible to create a world with little use for prisons because there are so few prisoners . . . where people get a chance, starting in early childhood, to deal with their life traumas in a therapeutic, healing way. We can choose to bring the finest schools to the very neighborhoods that used to be considered the most crime ridden. We can teach not just reading, writing, and arithmetic, but also the calculus of how to function in an increasingly complex and multilayered society.

We should decriminalize drugs and take the billions spent on our inane "drug war" and funnel it into treatment and prevention. Remember, drugs wouldn't cost that much if they weren't illegal. It's the black market that makes them expensive and creates the dangerous subculture of drug crime. Right now, all that is a pipe dream, pun intended.

When an alcoholic gets sober, he must replace the booze with something more than water. He must give himself new rewards. Similarly, to reduce crime, America needs to offer criminals a better alternative! The criminal needs to be able to get what he wants—money, status, self-esteem—through legal, legitimate means.

We need to clear an alternative path for these underclass youth—both inner city and rural; black, white, and Hispanic—so that they're not a crime statistic waiting to happen. We must focus, like a laser beam, on this subclass of neglected, marginally educated youth who are institutionalized, first in bad schools, then in prisons. We must level the playing field to give these young people a better shot at avoiding crime, gangs, and drugs by counteracting their toxic upbringings with a first-rate education that heals them as it teaches them. Only this will break the cycle of intergenerational crime.

The most important changes need to happen in American homes and in our neighborhoods. How many of us feel that we would be better people today had we only gotten more unconditional love, more affection, more attention, and more guidance? The path to a healthier, happier, more law-abiding community lies, first and foremost, in the hands of parents. Parents who are dysfunctional because of the pain of their own childhood traumas need to seek psychological help. Parents who are alcoholic or drug addicted need to get into recovery. Parents who are abusive need to be confronted.

Perhaps the most important first step in freeing ourselves from our dependence on incarceration is to start thinking about all the Americans who are locked up! As you walk around every day, cherish your freedom and ask yourself, *What can I do to help those who are unfairly treated by our justice system?* You may find yourself unable to put them out of your mind. Then you will surely do something.

Chapter Eight
THE BREEDERS: Addicted to Procreation

Tuesday, March 17, 2009, is a date that will live in tabloid infamy. It was nighttime, in a modest suburb outside Los Angeles, when Nadya Suleman returned home from the hospital with the first two of her eight newborns. She'd left six preemies behind at the hospital, all severely underweight and attended to by an army of doctors and nurses. Inside the home, her six other young kids were waiting for Mommy's return. So, let's do the math: two infants in the SUV, plus six preemies in the hospital, plus six tots waiting at home. The grand total? Fourteen children.[1] The infamous OCTOMOM had arrived, having artificially inseminated herself onto the world stage.

The media went nuts. A pack of paparazzi descended on Nadya's SUV as it pushed through a huge crowd of curiosity seekers, neighbors, and mainstream press. The frenzy grew as it became apparent Nadya planned to pull into her garage and roll down the door, potentially depriving the "pap" swarm a shot of the infants. It quickly turned into a stampede as photographers jumped on the SUV, riding it right into the garage with a hoard of gawkers on their heels. Nadya's handlers frantically tried to shut the garage door, which was dented in the process.[2] I covered the babe-in-arms circus on *Issues.*

VELEZ-MITCHELL: It turns out Octomom saw this chaos. She called the cops. Here is her 911 call while she's trapped in the garage swarmed by paparazzi, courtesy of radaronline.com.

(911 CALL TRANSCRIPT)

NADYA SULEMAN, MOTHER OF OCTUPLETS: Hi, yes, this is—ok, my name is Nadya Suleman. I'm coming back to come to my house. I'm picking up two of my eight babies. The paparazzi is dangerous. They're trying to break up the garage door. We've pulled in here and they're swarming the whole area. I need help.

MIKE WALTERS, ASSIGNMENT MANAGER, TMZ: My favorite part of this whole thing . . . she refers to herself as Octomom for the first time. She actually says, "What am I, the president?" As everyone banged on the car she then says, "Here she go, Octomom's going to call 911 again."[3]

America ran smack into the Octomom at the intersection of two of our most persistent cultural addictions: celebrity and procreation! Like a growing number of celebrities, Nadya's fame was not the result of any useful accomplishment or display of talent. Her fame was of the carnie freak-show variety. And with every passing hour, the public's perception of her was turning increasingly sour. Initially, the octuplets' arrival had been greeted with the mindlessly fawning media coverage that seems to attend every megabirth. But the coverage pulled a 180 as the world learned that Nadya was unemployed, getting food stamps, owed $50,000 in student loans, and had been living with her parents, who had recently declared bankruptcy.[4] Then we found out she conceived her octuplets knowing full well that three of her older kids are disabled.[5] The tsk-tsking turned to outright denunciation when articles began appearing suggesting the octuplets' long and extremely expensive stay in the neonatal intensive-care unit of the hospital would likely be picked up by tax-payers, through Medi-Cal, California's healthcare program for the poor.[6]

People were astounded that Suleman had ever finagled a way to pay for the expensive artificial-insemination procedures that resulted in all fourteen children. Then we learned she had gotten $165,000 in disability payments after being injured in a riot at a state mental hospital where she had worked several years earlier.[7] And there was even more disgust as Octomom was accused of selling access to the kids to media and entertainment outlets. Not that anyone was all that shocked. What else are you supposed to do when you have fourteen hungry mouths to feed, no husband, and no job? *Issues* viewers were transfixed by this freaky mutation of a family.[8]

MIKE WALTERS, TMZ ASSIGNMENT MANAGER: Look, it's gone overboard and I'll tell you . . . talk about the babies being traumatized . . . cameras inside of the nursery while they're trying to eat.

VELEZ-MITCHELL: When you told me the photographer wanted to take a photograph of the diaper being changed it was like, I almost got sick, seriously.[9]

But, while we may feel oh-so-justified in attacking the Octo-mom, we should also come clean and admit she is but an extreme example of our cultural addiction to procreation. America has a split personality when it comes to procreation. Intellectually, we realize that many of our most intractable problems—from poverty to pollution—stem from the fact that there are just too many people using too few resources. However, on an emotional level, we glorify, romanticize, and encourage super-large families on reality shows, in movies, and on commercials.

Cheaper by the Dozen—Really?

America had about 76 million people in 1900.[10] We recently passed the 300 million mark. Do we really grasp the enormity of that? Our nation's population has more than tripled in less than one century! This is part of a catastrophic global trend. The world's population has jumped from 2.5 billion in 1950 to almost 6 billion in 1998.[11]

"Britney Spears's first album sold more copies than the Beatles's *Abbey Road*. That to me says: *Okay, there are too many people on earth.*"

—Becky Heineke, blogger at
overpopulationblog.blogspot.com

In the terrifying book *Beyond Malthus,* which documents a slew of calamitous repercussions resulting from our world's population explosion, the authors point out, "There has been more growth in population since 1950 than during the 4 million preceding years since our early ancestors first stood upright."[12] Estimates are the world's population will hit 9 billion by 2050. Planet Earth simply cannot sustain that kind of population growth. So, for our own survival, we need to take a good, hard look at why so many of us are addicted to having very large broods. Please understand, this is not a criticism of the natural desire to parent or the legitimate desire to have a family of a reasonable size. We're talking about people who are going to extremes.

Craving Kids

What does it mean to be addicted to procreation? It means having babies for the same reasons people drug or overeat . . . to escape from painful feelings and to fill a void. Nadya is the poster child for this phenomenon. She admits that she got pregnant repeatedly to heal the trauma she experienced growing up in what she described as a "dysfunctional" home as an only child who felt isolated. "That was always a dream of mine, to have a large family, a huge family, and—I just longed for certain connections and attachments with another person that I, I really lacked, I believe, growing up (as an only child)," Nadya told NBC's Ann Curry.[13] That justification for having a child, or fourteen in this case, can also be described as "using" a child or children to work out emotional and psychological issues.

"From a psychoanalytic view, there can be a deep emptiness inside and the emptiness gets filled by feeling the fantasy and the idealization of motherhood. The fantasy is that 'I will now be loved.' First when you are pregnant it is 'I am full,' and secondly, when I have these children then I will be loved and they will belong to me. No one, on another level psychodynamically, will ever leave me."

—Dr. Judy Kuriansky, radio host
and professional therapist

Emotional trauma should be worked out on a therapist's couch or in a Twelve Step program for codependency, not in a fertility clinic. Nadya says she suffered depression after a divorce that she believes was brought on by her inability to have children the old-fashioned way.[14] What she should have realized is that depression signals a void on the inside that needs to be fixed from the inside . . . and by that I don't mean with an insemination.

Like all addiction, our drug of choice, be it booze or babies, never gives us the long-term results we're seeking. When Nadya didn't get that sought-after sense of "attachment" after having half a dozen kids, it should have been clear that she was not going to fill her emptiness by having eight more. She should have figured out that no amount of kids could ever complete her. But, to remodel that now tired Twelve Step cliché, insanity is doing the same thing fourteen times and expecting a different result. Nadya may have envisioned herself in a real-life version of *The Waltons*, but she ended up starring in a reality show so freaky it played out mostly as sporadic installments on Internet gossip sites.

"People have children for many reasons. Unfortunately, most of them are the wrong ones: because they don't believe in contraception, to show their parents how it is supposed to be done, or to create their own little cheerleading section that will love them unconditionally. When you look at our overburdened foster-care and adoption system, and all the children waiting to be adopted, you really have to wonder what people are thinking."

—Anne McIntyre, single, childless business executive

Natural Urge or Neurotic Impulse?

Like most addictive issues, the litmus test is the intention—the motive in picking up the addictive substance or behavior. *Am I drinking to get blind drunk? Am I getting pregnant to distract myself and blot out uncomfortable feelings?* Experts point to a slew of neurotic reasons for having children:

- to get a sense of purpose and identity
- to ease loneliness and isolation

- to assuage feelings of abandonment
- to compensate for insecurity, self-consciousness, and social anxiety through a cute sidekick/accessory
- to get attention from the child as well as adults
- to indulge in untreated codependency
- to try to see what you looked like as a kid
- to fit in and gain the acceptance of others who also have children
- to try to save a marriage or a relationship
- to prove one's sexual potency and fertility (virility for men)
- to try to establish evidence of heterosexuality if experiencing internal conflicts over sexual orientation or in the closet
- to prove one's intelligence or beauty as reflected in offspring
- to get money from the government or another party
- to have power and ownership over another human being
- to achieve a preconceived notion of the ideal family size

If the root cause of the psychological or emotional problem is not addressed, the procreation addict will seek another kid fix, as the first child grows up and becomes independent. Says Beverly Hills psychiatrist Dr. Carole Lieberman, "The mom may feel abandoned and act quickly to fill the void again with a new baby who will reply upon her and her partner and define their lives."[15]

So what is a spiritually sound reason to conceive? How about a motive centered on love. Having a child can be a profound expression of the love that exists between two human beings.

"What is the right reason to procreate? A desire to give . . . a healthy desire to nurture something."

—Dr. Judy Kuriansky, author of
The Complete Idiot's Guide to a Healthy Relationship

Get a Life

Ideally, you should have a life to share with your child, as opposed to expecting that your child will give your life meaning. Yet "I live for my kids" is a common refrain from parents. Wow, what enormous pressure on a kid to have to be someone else's *raison d'être*.

Ironically, it's likely to cause the child to resent the parent as the child is likely to feel suffocated by and enmeshed with the parent who is living through the kid. That is classic codependency. Or, in other words, the addiction to being "needed." It should be noted that you can be an addict and a codependent at the same time. It's called a "double winner."

So What if I Want a Big Family . . .
Mind Your Own Business

This is the common refrain of many Americans who consider family size a personal lifestyle choice that is nobody else's business but their own. China may have a one-child-only rule that is perceived as repressive and cruel, but Americans have the freedom to be *Jon and Kate Plus 8* or have nineteen kids like the Duggars, featured on national television. While I'm certainly not suggesting the U.S. government imitate China and create laws restricting how many children we can have, what I am saying is that we need to own up to the inherent irresponsibility of having large numbers of children without any consideration of the impact on the world around us.

My dad used to say, "Freedom isn't the right to shout fire in a crowded movie theater." Perhaps that should be revised to "Freedom isn't the right to pop out a football team and then put them on television with the excuse that you need to make money to feed them." If you think a massive brood is a harmless curiosity, perhaps this stat will snap you out of denial. The United States population is expected to soar from 309 million to at least 419 million by 2050! That's about 110 million more people in four decades.[16]

Too Many with Too Much

Americans actually have a greater moral responsibility than the rest of the world to be judicious about procreating. Why? According to the United Nations, a child born in the industrial world consumes and pollutes more over his or her lifetime than do dozens of children born in developing countries.[17] That's because kids in developing countries don't get closets full of designer clothes, garages full of toys, dozens of birthday gifts, and a mountain of video games. Also, I don't think they have Chuck E. Cheese's in Bangladesh! Because of our overindulgent lifestyle, environmentalists estimate having one child in the United States is equal to having at least forty kids in a developing country! So, Mr. Duggar, your having nineteen kids in America is like having 760 kids in Africa or India.

Population Control Is Perplexing

There is some good news on America's population-control front. It should be pointed out that many Americans are opting for fewer children. The average size of the American family is near an all-time low of about 3.2 humans.[18] Our fertility rate is slightly below 2.1 children per woman, which is the replacement rate.[19] Sounds like it's under control, right?

But other stats seem to completely contradict that. In 2007, American women gave birth to more than 4 million infants, the most ever![20] Here's one key to the puzzle: more than 25 percent of those babies were born to women having their third or fourth child![21] In other words, what we're seeing is a divergence, with increasing numbers of American women choosing fewer children or no children, but a crucial segment of the population opting for big families. With a population of 300 million and counting, that sizable chunk of women opting for large families is one reason the population is expected to keep spiking.

I realize this is a sensitive and emotional subject. Many Americans come from large families and cherish the experience of growing up with three, four, or even more siblings. As adults, they often seek to replicate what feels comfortable and natural to them. Pointing out the very real problems of overpopulation should not be perceived as a condemnation. History is filled with ever-changing circumstances that have always required humans to embrace new ways of thinking—if only for their own survival.

The continued population boom in the United States is also being fueled by what's called "population momentum." Even a population like ours, which is at or below replacement-level fertility, will keep growing. Why? Because the higher fertility—in our nation's recent past—produced more babies. Those babies have now matured and are currently making babies. So it can take a few generations for the population to stabilize and lower, even if the average woman is having fewer kids than her mom or grandma. It's like turning around a big, gray battleship. Population trends don't turn sharply downward overnight without something horribly catastrophic occurring, such as famine, an epidemic of disease, or genocide.

"The diseases are just going to get worse. They are evolving as we are evolving. A disease could arise which we do not have immunity to, and in our interconnected world, we have contact with so many people and things are spread so easily, lots of people could die. It could be a self-regulation of Mother Nature. We think we are the only organisms on this planet, but we're not. We're in balance with everything else here, and at some point the balance is going to tip too far and we are going to get the bad end of the deal."

—Becky Heineke, blogger at overpopulationblog.blogspot.com

Another obvious reason for the United States population boom is that Americans are living longer. In 2001, life expectancy at birth for the total population reached a record high of about seventy-seven years, up from about seventy-five years in 1990.[22]

Immigration is yet another reason we can expect our population to keep expanding. Between now and 2050, the Hispanic population is expected to triple. *USA Today* reports, "Even if immigration is limited, Hispanics' share of the population will increase because they have higher birth rates than the overall population. That's largely because Hispanic immigrants are younger than the nation's aging baby boom population."

Another huge factor is religion. Hispanics, whether immigrant or American born, are overwhelmingly Roman Catholic. The church still shuns artificial birth control, preaching that sex is a sin unless it's done within the context of marriage, retaining "its intrinsic relationship to the procreation of human life." Catholic Church doctrine condemns "Any action which either before, at the moment of, or after sexual intercourse, is specifically intended to prevent procreation—whether as an end or as a means." Abstinence during certain times of a woman's cycle is allowed as it takes advantage of "a faculty provided by nature."[23]

If there's one thing I've learned, it's not to argue religion at the dinner table, or even in a book like this. However, perhaps because I'm Puerto Rican and Irish (and my bosses assumed I was doubly Catholic), I was often sent to cover Pope John Paul II during my decades as a TV news reporter. I viewed these religious assignments as fun, out-of-town jaunts. So I never told my assignment editors that my parents were lapsed Catholics who preferred to dabble in Reichian therapy and Zen Buddhism while neglecting to have me baptized. The upshot is, while my mom and dad never attended Mass, I did . . . lots of times . . . on the clock as a reporter. I followed the late Pope as he visited Mexico and saw—with my own eyes— the enormous sway he held over the masses there. His word was taken as gospel by many millions in Latin America who follow church teachings unquestioningly. And the message was clear: make more babies, apparently even if you can't afford to feed them.

It's not just Catholicism. Most religions seem hardwired to promote procreation, perhaps—in part—as a form of self-preservation. While the Catholic Church apparently feels its principles are above and beyond questions of demographics and population, I know the Church does address the issue of human suffering. I believe much of the human suffering going on today is caused by the fact that we simply have too many humans beings born into a world that doesn't want them, doesn't appear to need them, and can't even feed them.

One Child Dies Every Five Seconds as a Result of Hunger![24]

While not big on organized religion, I am a huge fan of Jesus Christ. I feel strongly that Jesus Christ would not be in favor of mass starvation. Suffice it to say that our cultural addiction to procreation is very much intertwined with a variety of religious doctrines whose roots stem way back to a time when the mere concept of billions of human beings was simply unfathomable. In the controversial book *Conversations with God*, the author purports to find himself in a two-way dialogue with the Almighty. He takes the opportunity to ask God why he doesn't solve problems like world hunger. He says God's reply is this: "The day YOU really want an end to hunger, there will be no more hunger. I have given you all the resources with which to do that."[25]

Whether you believe he was talking to God or not, the truth is obvious. Ending world hunger is up to us—you and me. The fact is, we let 700 children die of hunger every hour; 16,000 children die of hunger every day.

Starvation is a slow and painful way to die. In our world today, most of these starvation victims are under the age of five. So many babies are coming into this world just to die. Is that a respect for life?

We are in denial. We pretend that these deaths are not happening and that we are "good people" as long as we can feed our own children. Unless it involves a massive hurricane or earthquake, these child-starvation deaths in faraway lands rarely attract news coverage or outside help. If you consider an innocent child dying of starvation to be an obscenity, then we've already hit bottom on our cultural addiction to procreation. There is a better way!

Adopt Me, Please

There are 145 million orphans in the world.[26] That's UNICEF's estimate. An orphan is defined as a child who has lost one or both parents. About 15 million children are double orphans, meaning they've lost both their mother and father. The vast majority of these orphans are in the developing world.[27]

Brangelina (Brad Pitt and Angelina Jolie) and Madonna may have made adoption trendy, but that doesn't mean it's a bad thing. Adoption, either of American children or children in a foreign land, is one obvious way to fulfill one's desire for parenthood—to nurture and give—and alleviate crushing social problems in the process. My therapist once said something that really impacted me: "You don't have to give birth to your own biological offspring to be a parent. You can be a parent to someone else's child or you can parent animals. You can even parent forests and oceans." I agree. We need to expand our circle of compassion beyond our own flesh and blood.

There is so much life out there that desperately needs nurturing. To do so is to be emotionally sober in a resource-starved world. To adopt an orphan or "parent" our neglected environment is also a way of making amends for the destruction we've inevitably wrought as a member of our materialistic culture. Making amends is a crucial part of a spiritual recovery from any addiction.

Dateline Niger

On May 4, 2010, I was reading the *New York Times* when I came upon the story of the famine in the West African nation of Niger. "Outside the state food warehouses here, women sift in the dirt for spilled grains of rice. Seven hundred miles to the east, mothers pluck bitter green berries and boil them for hours in an attempt to feed their children." I was about to bite into some morning toast but lost my appetite as I went on to read about how 12 percent of Niger's children are "acutely malnourished,"[28] with skinny arms that reach out for any morsel of food. But my sadness soon turned to frustration. Niger, while one of the poorest countries in the world, has the highest birthrate in the world! My frustration turned to rage as I read that there's little family planning in this Muslim country. One woman who was boiling leaves in the hopes of making them edible had a brood of seven children. Another frantic mother had five kids. Ten children is not uncommon. This is standard operating procedure all over the developing world. Niger's fertility rate is a mind-boggling 7.68 children per woman. Compare that to Japan's fertility rate of 1.20.[29]

Join the Pop Corps

There are many Americans making extraordinary efforts and pumping many millions into fighting hunger, poverty, and disease in Africa—and the rest of the developing world. It's admirable. Still, I can't help but wonder why it isn't completely obvious that the first and foremost objective and focus of all international humanitarian work must be population control. Overpopulation is the underlying problem and the common thread that runs through all of the other social problems, like malnutrition and disease. Since population can grow exponentially, especially in a place like Niger, preventing one birth is potentially preventing a thousand or even a million down the road.

We spend many millions fighting diarrhea, malaria, and measles. Wouldn't it make more sense to focus on reducing the number of humans through birth control so there are fewer people in the risk pool for those diseases? Of course, this is best illustrated by the AIDS pandemic.

The number of people infected by AIDS is growing by almost 3 million every year! Right now, about 33 million people are believed to be infected around the world.[30] For every 100 people put on treatment, 250 are newly infected. In Uganda alone, American money keeps about 200,000 people on AIDS treatment.[31] Still, our generosity cannot keep up with the spread of the epidemic.

Pouring money into birth control and family planning would automatically reduce the number of people born with AIDS and the number of people who might develop it during their lifetimes. Population control should be the first line of defense and the top priority. But preventing disease or death by preventing a person from existing isn't as dramatic as allowing someone to be born and then contract a disease from which they need to be cured. The absence of a person is an abstract concept. Abstract concepts are not as politically or socially enticing as living, breathing problems. Simply put, it's hard to take credit for saving a person who never was.

It's no longer an option to say, "Well, overpopulation is happening in other countries, so it's their problem, not mine." We are all sharing an ever-dwindling chunk of the earth's precious resources, so an unwanted, preventable pregnancy is going to impact all of us, whether it occurs in Somalia or Santa Fe.

Even if we made population control priority number one, how could we overcome the intense cultural resistance in much of the developing world to family planning, birth control—including the Pill—and condoms? One counterintuitive way is to reduce infant mortality in those countries. In the book *How Many People Can the Earth Support?* author Joel Cohen quotes experts who say, "No population in the developing world has experienced a sustained fertility reduction without first having gone through a major decline in infant and child mortality."[32] It would seem that many parents have a lot of children on the assumption that some will die. When children become more likely to survive, then parents are forced to rethink the equation and make long-term plans for health care and education. That's when the impracticality of a very large family becomes more obvious.

The Future Is Female

Perhaps the most effective way to change the mind-set that results in too many children is to free the minds of the women having those children. In *Beyond Malthus,* the authors write, "In every society for which data are available, the more education women have, the fewer children they have. In Egypt, for example, 56 percent of women with no schooling became mothers while still in their teens, compared with just 5 percent of women who remained in school past the primary level."[33]

Women who are educated realize they have other options beyond the role of wife and mother. They often delay having children to pursue those options, establishing a career or following a passion, be it art, business, or public service. They are also less inclined to have children for fear-based reasons, such as wanting a safety net in old age. Conversely, in highly patriarchal societies where women are subjugated, controlled, and not allowed power over their ability to procreate, birthrates are soaring.

Frankly, if we hope to survive as a species, the future better be female . . . or at least centered on matriarchal values and respect for women and girls. This is where American women come in. We are the most powerful nation on earth, and about half of us are female. American women are arguably among the most empowered women on the planet, with most of us feeling that we are in control and in charge of our capacity to reproduce, or not, as we see fit.

In recovery programs, Step Twelve occurs when, after having a spiritual awakening ourselves, we carry the message to others who are still suffering. Spreading the word is called "twelve-stepping." It really is up to us American women to twelve-step the developing world when it comes to reproductive sobriety.

There are two messages that we have to get out: you do not have to get pregnant because you can use birth control, and you should not get pregnant if you don't have the ability to provide for that child's financial and emotional well-being from the moment of its birth well into the future. Adhering to just these two rules would preclude many of the pregnancies in the world today. Experts estimate that, in the developing world, one birth in four is unwanted. As for intentional pregnancies, a leading cause is said to be the procreators' desire for a large family. American women can offer proof to women in the developing world that smaller families equal greater freedom. Train wrecks like the Octomom should be used as a cautionary tale.

While poverty and disease should make people in developing countries think twice before procreating, America has its own brand of struggles with thoughtless and irresponsible procreation.

True story: In New York State a cocaine-addicted, unemployed, and homeless woman gives birth to a baby, who is placed in foster care. The woman proceeds to give birth to three more children. Each infant tests positive for cocaine. Each baby is quickly taken from the mother and put in foster care. The last baby is taken from the mother a week after its birth. The judge overseeing this woman's case becomes fed up, noting, "It is painfully obvious that a parent who has already lost to foster care all four of her children born over a six-year period, with the last one having been taken from her even before she could leave the hospital, should not get pregnant again soon, if ever. This is a practical, social, economic and moral reality." The judge added that the babies were "for all practical purposes motherless and fatherless." Calling that unacceptable, the judge then ruled that this mother could not become pregnant again until she proved that she was capable of taking care of the kids she'd already brought into this world. Ditto for the dad! Unconstitutional? Probably![34] But I bet you can understand the judge's frustration.

Welfare advocates have fashioned a system that—albeit unintentionally—encourages many young, uneducated, unemployed mothers to get pregnant in order to receive the additional government check that comes with each new, hungry mouth. They call it "IQC" or "Increase for a Qualified Child." Some people call it "going on the county." While welfare reform has achieved some improvements, we—as a culture—need to devise a more sophisticated system that protects children while ending financial incentives that spur young women to get pregnant for the worst of reasons.

Family planning must be part of the curriculum in public school. We need more innovative programs, like the great one I read about where girls are given a taste of the rigors of parenthood by having to take care of a "mock" baby for a month. The concept of "abstinence only" needs to be exposed for the false notion that it is. We need to get real and accept that intellectual concepts like abstinence are a very low defense against powerful biological urges, especially among hormonal teens. As Americans who pride ourselves on helping others, we need to get our own "house in order" so that we may carry the message to others.

The Politics of Procreation Makes Very Strange Bedfellows

The Catholic Church, welfare proponents, and Hollywood are all complicit in overpopulation. Every baby born is a new customer for movie-inspired merchandise from SpongeBob SquarePants lunch boxes to Hannah Montana designer wear. Cable networks are also getting monstrously huge ratings following freakishly large families like the Gosselins, the Duggars, and—though she's yet to score her own major show—Octomom. There are forty children between the three families.

Gay Is the New Green?

It's ironic. For most of human history people needed to procreate persistently to survive as a species. But, today, we've reached a tipping point. Now, overpopulation is the biggest threat to our survival as a species (not to mention all the other species we're taking down with us). What solution would you prefer to restore balance? A plague? Another world war?

Nature invariably comes up with solutions to problems that spring up in the environment. The "carrying capacity" of any species is the number of individuals a given environment can sustain. This is Mother Nature in her most efficient form. If the population of any species gets to be too much, nature has a bag of tricks to help control things. It is interesting that the world's gay-rights movement is surging at the very moment in history when our global population is soaring. Is nature providing balance by offering an alternative for coupling that precludes procreation in its traditional form and even encourages adoption? It's just something to think about.

More Does Not Equal Better

There is a pop-culture term for people who are obsessed with procreation. Some call them "breeders." That term was taken from the business of animal breeding where animal exploiters breed dogs, cats, and horses for profit, ignoring the fact they are contributing to a massive pet overpopulation crisis. Many millions of these beautiful animals are killed every year because there are simply not enough homes for them. Our all-American, more-is-better mentality is a form of madness that often results in cruelty to both four- and two-legged creatures.

Reducing Every American's Carbon Footprint

If Americans want to continue to have the freedom to create big families, then we have a moral obligation to compensate by tempering our voracious consumption of finite resources. We cannot keep indulging all of our cultural addictions simultaneously! Experts warn that, given the world's surging population, food production is going to have to skyrocket or mass starvation will soon become as commonplace as floods or fires. We have a moral obligation to reform food production so it can feed the most people using the fewest resources.

Many Americans are surprised to learn they can take a huge leap in reducing their slice of the earth's resource pie by simply going vegetarian or, better yet, vegan. According to the United Nations, "More than half of the world's crops are used to feed animals, not people." It takes over seven pounds of grain to create one pound of edible hog flesh. That same amount of grain could feed an entire family for a week in a Third World country. Each year, we could feed the entire United States and still have enough food left over to feed 1 billion people if we simply gave up meat and switched to a plant-based diet. Yet, when we talk about the earth's dwindling resources and how the world's exploding population is causing a starvation crisis, the simple, obvious solution of forgoing meat and dairy is rarely mentioned! Very few mainstream environmental organizations even have vegetarian platforms. Why not? Because many so-called environmentalists, including Al Gore, are still carnivores. While eager to tell everyone else how to live, they—themselves—refuse to alter their own most ingrained habits, like meat consumption. The idea of Al chatting up some fellow VIP about global warming over steak and eggs is, to my mind, the perfect portrait of hypocrisy. And then there's water.

Water, Water Everywhere and Not a Drop to Drink!

The greatest threat to people trapped in a vortex of overpopulation is the absence of clean, drinkable water. Lawrence Smith, president of the Population Institute, notes, "If the water goes, the species goes. That sounds kind of alarmist considering there's water all around us, but 97 percent plus is saltwater, and the freshwater that we use to sustain ourselves is just native to 3 percent. . . . So the accessibility of water, the competition for water, the availability of water is going to be a major, major threat."[35]

Let it be noted that it takes hundreds of times more water to make meat than it does vegetables and grains. It takes about 60 gallons of water to produce a pound of potatoes versus at least 2,500 gallons to produce a pound of meat. In fact, some experts say it may take more than twice that.[36] While some quibble with the exact numbers because there are many variables, nobody disputes that meat production is phenomenally more water intensive than vegetables and grains, including soybeans, rice, wheat, and corn.

Put another way, the water that goes into a 1,000-pound cow could fill a harbor. So skip the burger if you want to feel better about putting a bun in the oven.

Smarter Choices

Whether it's food or families, it's become imperative that we all start making more evolved choices that take into consideration the impact on our environment and the other people/creatures with whom we share this finite, fragile earth. Imagine a world without overpopulation. It's a world where every child has a home and food to eat. It's a world with no lonely, traumatized orphans. It's a world where all the people alive share our collective resources in a fair manner so that global warming has been abated. It's a world where every human and animal gets the attention, sustenance, and nurturing they need. Some would call that a naïve fantasy. But to make any profound change, we must first let go of old thinking and set a new intention. Why don't we close our eyes and, for a few seconds, try to imagine this kinder world.

Let's make it easier for couples, both straight and gay, to adopt. Let's have the courage to teach family planning in schools. Let's get our own house in order: eat responsibly, procreate responsibly, show compassion, and reach out to help other nations struggling with overpopulation. Let's give birth to a new consciousness.

Chapter Nine
THE GLUTTONS: Addicted to Food

————————————

I headed for the refrigerator one evening when my ninety-four-year-old mother looked at me from across the kitchen. She sized me up and then quietly said, "Jane, you're getting FAT." Now, my mother doesn't criticize me very often so this got my attention. Of course, I was irritated. Who wants to be told the truth about something like that! But it was the kind of thing only somebody who loves you would dare to say. Call it a one-sentence intervention. It did the trick. It was precisely what I needed to break through the logjam of my denial. It had been a while since my scale had died. I never replaced the battery. My fear of finding out how much I weighed was so ingrained in my psyche that I went to the store twice to buy a new battery for my scale and got the wrong size each time.

What would Freud say?

Yes, I—like most Americans—have food issues. I never did while I was drinking. So long as I had my chardonnay security blanket, I could nibble on a salad and be perfectly content. But when that was taken away from me a decade and a half ago, suddenly food entered my life as a serious contender for my attention and my extremely addictive tendencies. It was my new route to escape!

At the age of fifty-four, I found it ever more difficult to keep the weight off. The days when I could run fifteen miles and take off five pounds in one afternoon of binge exercise were long gone. Although I do sweaty yoga, which I find extraordinarily strenuous, I seemed to be compensating for it afterward with sweet treats I felt I had earned. Along with my food addiction, I discovered there are subsets, including sugar addiction. I am a sugar addict. I also have a tendency to be a "night eater." It appears, despite all my years of recovery and therapy, I still have some real emotional issues. I was eating to stuff down feelings and conflicts that used to disappear in the fog of alcohol.

Why do I tell you all this? Because you're not going to listen to anything I have to say if I don't first prove to you that I understand what food cravings feel like and how powerful they are. In recovery lingo, it's called "qualifying." And, believe me, I qualify.

Millions of Americans can relate. We have been self-medicating ourselves with fat and sugar for so long it has become a standard of living. As a result, our country is suffering from a mind-blowing obesity crisis. Two-thirds of Americans are overweight or obese.[1] It would be safe to say that obesity is our nation's biggest health issue, and reports show this epidemic impacts every facet of our lives from health care to global warming. We're fat! Our kids are fat! And it's making us miserable, sick, unattractive, and costing us a fortune. So . . . WTF are we going to do about this problem of ours?

"I've been in practice for thirteen years, and when I first started out I had mostly healthy-weight kids with a few obese kids that I would see. Now the opposite seems to be true. I have mostly overweight and obese patients and a few that are normal weight patients."

—Dr. Leslie Brown, pediatrician

Look for a moment at this behavior from the perspective of addiction. It's easy to admit the obvious. We are a nation obsessed with food. On April 25, 2010, in the *New York Times Book Review*, *most* of the books on the advice and how-to list were about food: *Women, Food and God*; *Home Cooking with Trisha Yearwood*; *Jamie's Food Revolution*; *The Kind Diet*; *The Pioneer Woman Cooks*; *Hungry Girl 1-2-3*; *Now Eat This!*; *Food Rules*; *The Belly Fat Cure*; *Cook This, Not That!*; *The New Atkins For a New You*; and my personal favorite, *Skinny Bitch*.

TV has also jumped on the food gravy train with an entire network devoted to food, plus a slew of shows on various networks that form the new genre dubbed "Fat TV": NBC's *The Biggest Loser*, A&E's *Kirstie Alley's Big Life*, Oxygen's *Dance Your Ass Off*, and Fox's *More to Love*.[2]

We're talking and thinking and watching shows about food and fat and, as we do, eating more and getting fatter. Ain't that the perfect portrait of addiction! By way of comparison, it reminds me of how I spoke incessantly about my alcohol problem for years with various therapists and friends. Even as I castigated myself, I kept drinking through the whole process. I rationalized that I was "working on it." Being an alcoholic, my drinking progressively got worse, despite my willingness to bore my friends with an endless litany of excuses and explanations that really should've been billable hours.

Unfortunately, as I know now, the kind of talk in which I was engaged was rife with alcoholic thinking. I was essentially negotiating with my disease and using my therapist and my friends as mediators. I was "bargaining" with my cravings, trying to come up with some deal that would allow me to have it both ways: get rid of my drinking problem while still drinking. It was about as effective as the Mideast peace process. It was only when I finally hit bottom and admitted to myself and to another human being that I was totally powerless over alcohol—helpless against even a drop of it—that the huge shift occurred and I was able to walk away from the stuff. I had surrendered to the truth. Sobriety, no matter what substance we're talking about—booze or food—demands, above all else, honesty and surrender!

Can we, as a nation, get honest about our relationship with food? Can we surrender to the truth and acknowledge we have become powerless over our cravings? Let's admit it's not about being big boned or having a slow metabolism or not having the time to cook. We're overweight—despite all the negative ramifications to our health, our appearance, and the environment—because we, as a nation, are culturally food addicted. Say it!

I am a food addict!

I am powerless over food! Tell it to a friend. And if you're living with somebody who's overweight or obese, confront them about it, just as you would if they had a drinking or drug problem. Don't dance around the big elephant in the room. Don't act like a golf journalist at a Tiger Woods news conference! Lovingly say the words. "You're obese! I'm worried about you."

Do a Fat Intervention

Admittedly, there are challenges to telling someone you think he or she is fat. The recipient of your honesty is liable to get very angry and/or hurt. All of society's messages encourage us to ignore the fat issue and pretend it doesn't exist. This can be described as cultural codependency and mass enabling. When an individual or organization deviates from this unspoken pact, all hell breaks loose.

Film director Kevin Smith of *Clerks* fame is undoubtedly a brilliant artist. He is also obese. He was flying Southwest Airlines from Oakland to Burbank and had booked two seats because "it's way more comfortable and I have enough money to do it." Then he decided to try and catch an earlier flight on standby. He lucked out. At least initially. He was sent in to fill an empty seat. One seat! That's when he says an airline employee approached and ordered him off the jet. Smith became enraged! "I'm legit! I've passed the stinkin' arm-rest test. And still the lady asks me to get up and come with her off the plane," he fumed on Twitter. "I can fit into a Southwest Airlines seat, this is the important part of the story," Smith added on his website podcast. The airline apologized, and Smith was allowed to board another flight later that day.

But did the very smart Kevin Smith take away the most important lesson from this experience? I don't think so. To me, he sounds like a man who is still defiant about his apparent addiction to food and living in his disease. To wit, he rationalizes, "I'm a fat man. I've grown up fat and there are varying degrees of fat . . . Look, I'm fat, yes. But like, am I . . . John Candy yet? No."[3] To me, that sort of sounds like a drunk who gets totally wasted at the office holiday party, but comforts himself that he still managed to keep his job. What if, instead, he had taken that embarrassing airline experience as a sign that his addiction to food was making his life unmanageable? What if he had used that humiliating episode as a wake-up call to say, "I think I've got a problem. I'm powerless over food and I need help." Wouldn't that ultimately have been a better outcome for his future?

Smith's response was in line with the very misguided fat-acceptance movement, whose leaders argue any criticism of their weight is hate speech. That's a very effective way of stifling criticism, but I don't buy that obesity is in the same category as race, gender, or sexual orientation. We don't choose our race, gender, or sexual orientation. But, with rare exceptions, we are responsible for our weight. And, as is true with drinking and drugs, taxpayers and corporations end up footing the bill for the food addict's out-of-control weight problem. The total cost of obesity has shot past $140 billion a year.[4] It's estimated that weight issues account for almost 10 percent of United States health expenditures. Billions are lost by corporations because of the overweight or obese employee's doctor's visits and restricted activity.[5]

How Do We *Get It*?

In recovery we talk about high bottoms and low bottoms. A "bottom" is the lowest place an addict reaches before he or she decides it's time to change. One friend of mine likes to say, "You've hit bottom when you stop digging." Some addicts have that moment of clarity relatively early, and they have a chance to turn their lives around before all hell's broken loose. That's a high bottom. Others lose almost everything before they get it: their job, their family, their home. That's a low bottom. Even lower are those who die from their addiction. Then it's a little too late to have a moment of clarity, and at your funeral, people will shake their heads and say, "He just never got it."

So how do we Americans "get it" and confront our food addiction? It probably helps to break down the issue into its component parts. America's food problem is multidetermined, meaning there are a host of different influencing factors. The root causes of an addiction can be genetic, environmental, emotional, psychological, physical, and—let's not forget—spiritual. Usually, it's a combination of all of the above. In order to combat an addiction, you must look at all of the causes. As much as people like to say, "Losing weight is easy! Just eat less and exercise more," it's nearly impossible for most people to change their eating habits. If it were easy, we wouldn't be stuck with this epidemic. That one-dimensional approach reminds me of the naive *normies* who always ask alcoholics, "Can't you just have one glass of wine with dinner?"

One Nation Overweight

Exactly how many people are killed because of our collective addiction to food and the resultant obesity is a subject of debate in the scientific community. Obesity has been cited as a contributing factor in anywhere between 100,000 and 400,000 deaths in the United States every year.[6] "Obesity is catching up to tobacco as the leading cause of death in America. If this trend continues it will soon overtake tobacco," Julie Gerberding said in 2004 when she was the director of the CDC (Centers for Disease Control and Prevention).[7] A battle over studies and statistics ensued. What makes it so complicated is that being overweight or obese is a contributing factor in so many different illnesses, including:

- Coronary heart disease
- Type 2 diabetes
- Cancer (endometrial, breast, and colon)
- Hypertension (high blood pressure)
- Dyslipidemia (high total cholesterol or high levels of triglycerides)
- Stroke
- Liver and gallbladder disease
- Sleep apnea and respiratory problems
- Osteoarthritis (degeneration of cartilage and underlying bone within a joint)
- Gynecological problems (abnormal menses, infertility)

Let's face it, being fat affects every single aspect of a person's life. So obesity's true impact is like a Rubik's Cube, very hard to figure out.

In our country, powerful commercial interests are always working to influence the debate. Their methods are often ingenious, to wit: "Where's the Beef?" and "Got Milk?" The food and agriculture lobbies are among the most powerful in Washington. Officials who point the finger at food-related industries—especially meat and dairy production—can become the subject of a campaign to discredit them. Politicians who vote against the food-agriculture behemoth can find themselves targeted as "un-American" or "radical" come re-election time.

"Thirty-one million kids eat school lunches. Much of what is served in schools is a commodity—by that I mean the government says: 'Ahh, the dairy prices are falling. Let's buy up cheese to help the farmer and let's give the cheese to kids to eat.' Cheeseburgers, cheese pizzas. Not because anyone thinks they need more cholesterol, but because the law right now says that if meat prices fall, the government buys up meat. If cheese prices fall, the government buys up cheese. They serve it in prisons, they serve it in hospitals, they serve it in schools. And that's the law. Even while we have people running the school program saying: 'This is too many calories. It's too much fat.' They are absolutely in a bind."

–Dr. Neal Barnard, founder and president of
Physicians Committee for Responsible Medicine

Obesogenic

Suffice it to say that the CDC is correct in saying America has become obesogenic, meaning the environment in the United States promotes the overeating of bad foods. Obesogenic! What a great way to buttonhole the issue of cultural food addiction. But here's the real shocker! The blame for our nation's toxic food environment can be laid directly at the door of the government. In a nightmarishly ironic twist, the very government that is waging a campaign against obesity is responsible for and encourages it!

Uncle Sam Makes Us Fat, Then Tells Us to Diet

Time magazine did a brilliant cover story called "Getting Real About the High Price of Cheap Food" explaining, "Americans spend less than 10% of their incomes on food, down from 18% in 1966.[8] Those savings begin with the remarkable success of one crop: corn. Corn is king on the American farm, with production passing 12 billion bushels annually, up from 4 billion bushels as recently as 1970. When we eat a cheeseburger, a Chicken McNugget, or drink soda, we're eating the corn that grows on vast, monocrop fields in Midwestern states like Iowa. . . . Over the past decade, the Federal Government has poured more than $50 billion into the corn industry, keeping prices for the crop . . . artificially low. That's why McDonald's can sell you a Big Mac, fries and a Coke for around $5."[9] Without government subsidies, estimates are the average hamburger would cost more than twice that amount.[10]

"I felt that I was addicted to food. Of course I was. How else do you get to 450 pounds? I would eat all the time. I would go through the fast food drive-though on the way home from work before I would eat dinner. I felt like I couldn't stop. I say it is a drug. It's the cheapest drug out there. That's what makes it so potent. You can pull off at any time and for one dollar you can get a double cheeseburger."

–*Danny Cahill, Winner of* The Biggest Loser

The American taxpayers are subsidizing the production of corn that agribusiness feeds to factory farm animals. "Factory farmed" refers to an industrial system that traps animals in a high-speed assembly line from birth to slaughter. In the United States, small family farms are being pushed out of business, giving way to massive animal factories where billions of animals endure tortured existences in extremely tight quarters, never seeing the light of day. Despite escalating moral, health, and environmental concerns, America's top priority always seems to be keeping food prices low, even though cheap food is precisely what is seducing us into overeating. The government's corn subsidies allow fast food corporations to churn out cheap burgers and fries, thereby encouraging their overconsumption. Without the government's collusion, those burgers would be way too expensive for the average consumer to binge on.

"Meat production is subsidized by the government and so is dairy, so it is cheaper for them to make a hamburger than a veggie burger."

—*Neal Barnard, M.D., clinical researcher
and author of* Breaking the Food Seduction

Our Enabler-in-Chief Is the U.S. Government!

Why on earth is the U.S. government fueling our obesity crisis at the very same time it spends our tax dollars to warn us about the dangers of obesity? That's crazy! Like a fox. Our politicians keep handing over these insidious, self-defeating farm subsidies because lawmakers, more than anything else, want to get re-elected. If they play along with the big industrial farmers, they get big donations. Conversely, any politician who tries to rewrite the farm bill to wipe out those subsidies knows that agribusiness will declare war on him and try to force him out of office. It's the vicious cycle of addiction, Washington style. Our government is a moral mess, with corporations basically controlling the very agencies that are supposed to regulate them. All addiction leads to cynicism and moral corruption.

I can hardly remember the last time I stepped foot in a fast food restaurant. When I did, I think it was only to use the ladies room, not to order anything. At my old job with *Celebrity Justice,* coworkers used to joke that I would rather find out my partner had gone into a topless bar than a fast food restaurant. It's true! Sadly, I don't have a lot of company on this. Every day, one-fourth of all Americans eat fast food![11] Like lemmings, Americans keep going to the killer trough, their blinders tightly fastened. Here's some of what these fast food addicts conspicuously ignored:

In 2004, the groundbreaking documentary *Super Size Me* put the problem in our face using an extraordinarily clever technique. We watched Morgan Spurlock get thicker and thicker and sicker and sicker as he subjected his body to a fast food–only diet. After only a month, he had gained almost twenty-five pounds and began to suffer liver dysfunction and depression. It took Morgan well over a year to get back to his normal weight.[12]

This was followed by the highly acclaimed dramatic film *Fast Food Nation* in 2006. Based on the best-selling nonfiction book of the same name, the film's tagline was "Do you want lies with that?" This film outlines how fast food production is not only gross, but involves the torture of factory farm animals while simultaneously dehumanizing those low-paid workers who have to slaughter them.[13]

Then in 2009 came the riveting documentary *Food, Inc.,* which—again—exposed the horrific cruelties of America's factory farms, where tightly packed cattle are forced to live in their own manure and where chickens are crammed into cages so small they can never stretch their wings. The film brilliantly outlines the health and environmental risks of factory farming, which is the pipeline to fast food. It proves to the viewer that industrial farming is unsustainable, meaning if we keep doing it much longer we're in for some heavy-duty blowback. Can you say salmonella?

In sum, you'd have had to be living under a supersized rock not to have heard all the loud warnings about fast food! Why then are Americans still spending well over $110 billion on fast food every year?[14] We spend more on fast food than on movies, books, magazines, newspapers, videos, and recorded music combined. Our increasingly overweight children often recognize fast food logos before they recognize their own name.

It's because we're addicts. Addicts do not respond to reason or rational argument. Do you think a heroin addict is going to quit shooting up just because you show the junkie a documentary about the dangers of heroin? Aw, but you can't compare food to heroin . . . YES, YOU CAN!

"The taste of sugar on the tongue releases opiates within the brain. You can demonstrate this on day one of life. If you have a newborn baby and need to take a drop of blood, the baby cries. Nurses learned a long time ago, if you take a little sugar water and you dribble it into a baby's mouth just before you do a heel stick the babies often don't cry—or they don't cry so much. Research shows there is sort of a pain killing effect with sugar."

–Dr. Neal Barnard, clinical researcher

I was disheartened to read that a group of scientists decided it would be a good idea to study rats to confirm the "addictive" properties of junk food. The research found that rats fed a high-fat, high-calorie diet—equivalent to fast food—developed compulsive eating habits, similar to a drug addiction. The study divided the rats into three groups. One group ate normal food, and the second was fed fatty foods for an hour a day. The third was fed fatty foods for up to twenty-three hours per day. Researchers reported that the third group began to eat compulsively, requiring more and more fatty food to get the same "high." They continued gorging even when threatened by electric shocks.[15]

Fast food overstimulates the "pleasure centers" in our head. Foods heavy in sugar and fat create "feel-good chemicals" that hit receptors. Those receptors react by demanding more, more, more. Also, just as word quickly spreads when a good party's going on, the number of these ravenous receptors grows. When countless hungry mouths inside your brain begin crying out for pleasure, that's called developing an addiction. So the body will now demand more and more sugary, fatty foods. It's a classic vicious cycle.

"We can make ourselves addicted to food . . . just by eating a lot of sugar. So if you are flooding your body with sugar, your receptors will change. Receptors, when they get empty, want more. It's like little mouths that want to be fed—like little kittens. And as you feed these little kittens, more kittens from the neighborhood come over . . . and more cats come to your house, and all of a sudden you've got more and more cats."

−Anne Katherine, author of
Lick It! Fix Her Appetite Switch

It's never quite enough. The researcher described the junk food rats this way: "They always went for the worst types of food, and as a result, they took in twice the calories as the control rats. When we removed the junk food and tried to put them on a nutritious diet— what we called the 'salad bar option'—they simply refused to eat. The change in their diet preference was so great that they basically starved themselves for two weeks after they were cut off from junk food . . . These same rats were also those that kept on eating (the junk food) even when they anticipated being shocked."[16] In other words, regardless of the pain and suffering it caused, the junk food was so like heroin that the regular healthy food ceased to offer any kind of pleasure rush by comparison. It might as well have been cardboard. Their mouths and their brains had become completely disinterested in anything but the fatty foods.

They really didn't need to torture a bunch of rats to figure that out. This is a perfect example of unnecessary animal experimentation. All you need to do is look at our kids! Millions of parents find it almost impossible to get their kids to eat any healthful foods, like green vegetables. I was at a friend's house for dinner once and saw a child actually start weeping when someone suggested he eat the vegetables on his plate. American kids are being turned into junk food junkies. And, once hooked, they're likely to remain that way the rest of their lives.

"Don't ever give a kid his first chicken nugget because if he doesn't know he likes it, he is not going to ask you to go there."

–Dr. Leslie Brown, pediatrician

Fast food makers intentionally overuse three highly addictive substances—fat, salt, and sugar—to ensure that customers will experience a craving for more fast food. Humans are genetically programmed to crave fat, salt, and sugar to get us through times of famine. But now, thanks to fast food, these three substances are being consumed in such excessive quantities that they're creating times of obesity. They're insidious because they kill our desire to eat anything healthful. Like those poor, exploited rats, we're likely to go for bad food or no food at all. After devouring greasy cheeseburgers and milkshakes on a regular basis, it's hard for a simple salad or an apple to even register with our dopamine receptors.

OA Can You See

They say food addiction is perhaps the hardest addiction to break because, unlike alcohol or drugs, every human being has to eat to live. So, every single day, we are confronted with our demon and must battle it out.

OA (Overeaters Anonymous) can help us eat in a sober way, developing a healthy relationship with food. If your food and/or sugar cravings feel overwhelming—physically or emotionally—the very best option would be for you to start going to OA meetings. They're easy to find. Just Google "Overeaters Anonymous." There are some interesting reasons Twelve Step programs like OA work when diets don't. Some are spiritual. Some are scientific.

"One of the paradoxes that causes people to be put in a trap is dieting. Dieting requires people to make an effort. You have to make yourself eat this way in the morning and you have to make yourself change to foods that are unfamiliar, and you have to take yourself out of the herd if your culture is food centered. These all cause effort. Any time we are making an effort we are causing our stress chemicals to flood the brain. So any time the stress chemicals build up in the eating center they will make a person eat. So a diet is a set up to eat. There isn't anyway to avoid that set up. This is why recovery in *Overeaters Anonymous* works with addiction when all the willpower in the world doesn't work. The very first step in all the 12 step programs is: I am powerless over this chemical. I admit I am powerless over this chemical and my life became unmanageable. By admitting powerlessness, it's the opposite of effort. It is letting

go. And when we let go we put that stress chemical, that 'effort'
chemical back in its box. Then something can change for us."

—Anne Katherine, licensed mental health counselor and author of
Anatomy of a Food Addiction: The Brain Chemistry of Overeating

I know exactly what Anne Katherine is talking about in the
above quote. For more than twenty years, I tried to use my
willpower to quit drinking. It never worked for more than a day or
so. But the first day I went into recovery and genuinely surrendered
to my powerlessness over alcohol, I felt a psychic shift and a relief
from cravings that I often describe as a miracle. I've come to find
out that there are biological underpinnings to that miracle. Surrender is the opposite of stress and effort. Surrender is the key.

Apply the Concept of Surrender
to Narrow the Food Battlefield

Unlike alcohol, we can't give up all food. So we have to manage
the gray areas. For example, we can surrender to being powerless
over the worst food. Try it! Surrender to the truth that you are powerless over fast food! Acknowledge that your willpower simply will
not work when trying to navigate the treacherous shoals of a fast
food menu filled with seductions like the Angus Third Pounder
(from McDonald's), which has between 720 and 860 calories and
about 39 grams of fat.[17] We know that willpower simply does not
work when applied to the substance to which you're addicted. So,
instead, surrender to the fact that you are powerless over the siren
call of fast food and see if you feel a sense of relief and strength.

Just as a recovering alcoholic will not drink even one drop of alcohol,
you must avoid even one bite of fast food. That one decision will eliminate a lot of the world's most intensely addictive foods. You can do this
one day at a time, which is how recovery works. Say, "Just for today I

will not visit a fast food restaurant." Say, "Just for today I will stop going through the drive-through lane of fast food joints." No excuses. Gradually, it will get easier. Then it will become second nature. One day, you won't even think about it. You will have found a new joy by discovering freedom from the cycle of bingeing and remorse.

If it helps, here's a fact likely to make even the most diehard fast food addict a little queasy. Today, the average hamburger has pieces of flesh from at least dozens to even hundreds of different cows. When you bite into that cheap burger, you're eating a lot of different creatures whose carcasses have been blended together.[18] Yuck!

Sugar, Sugar

In sobriety we talk about avoiding "people, places, and things" that can trigger our addiction. We just covered "places." Now it's time for "things." And when it comes to food, a big "thing" is sugar.

A while back, I admitted that, along with being a recovering alcoholic, I am also a sugar addict. I finally surrendered to the fact that I am powerless over sugar. A lot of recovering alcoholics are sugar addicts because there is so much sugar in alcohol, and when you remove the cocktail or wine, the craving for the sugar remains. Fifteen years after I had my last drink, my cravings for sugar had gotten out of hand, becoming harder and harder to control, and causing me to gain weight. I was learning, yet again, that all addiction is progressive.

"It feeds on itself. You get depressed. I was so depressed. It's a big spiral. When I got to be that big and that far gone—I was up over 450 pounds at one point—I felt like I was literally in a hole I couldn't get out of."

–*Danny Cahill, winner of* The Biggest Loser

I had already tried half measures, like switching to "natural" sugars such as maple syrup, agave nectar, and evaporated cane juice. But in recovery they say half measures avail us nothing. I had simply switched from cakes loaded with processed sugar to equally fattening cakes loaded with natural sugar. I finally had to let go of sugar . . . period . . . in all its forms . . . one day at a time. Now, when I'm having a sugar craving, I pray . . . and wait it out. I also eat naturally sweet fruits, like nectarines, cherries, bananas, and mangos. I make delicious desserts just with fruits. My other safety valve is stevia, which is a naturally sweet alternative to artificial sweeteners and also has virtually no calories. It even comes in packets like sugar. Of course, because it's so healthy and natural, this fantastic product is usually not available in regular supermarkets. You can get it at a health food store, a food co-op, or Whole Foods.

"Nobody ever went to the 7-11 at 9 o'clock at night to buy strawberries. Nobody ever went out to the grocery store at 11 o'clock at night because we just had to get cauliflower or green beans or tofu. What we tend to want is sugar or things that turn to sugar like starchy foods."

–Neal Barnard, M.D., clinical researcher and
author of Breaking the Food Seduction

Another Way to Narrow the Food Battlefield Is to Go Vegan

Vegans do not eat any meat or dairy products. The philosophy is simple and based on respect for the fellow creatures who share our world. Vegans believe animals are not ours to eat (or wear . . . or torture). People may give up meat and dairy for ethical, health, or spiritual reasons. I went vegan for all three.

The China Study is a powerhouse book about one of many studies that show a vegetarian diet is healthier and naturally lower in calories, fat, and cholesterol. The in-depth survey of lifestyle and disease in rural China and Taiwan found "People who ate the most animal-based foods got the most chronic disease . . . People who ate the most plant-based foods were the healthiest and tended to avoid chronic disease. These results could not be ignored," according to author Dr. T. Colin Campbell.[19]

I've been vegan for about fourteen years, and God only knows how fat or sick I'd be today if I hadn't made that leap. Going vegan was one of the very best decisions I've ever made in life, right up there with getting sober. In fact, you could call veganism food sobriety. Why? Sobriety is all about living a life of honesty, integrity, humility, and kindness. It's the antithesis of addictive behavior, which is self-centered, shortsighted, and often mean-spirited.

All addiction wreaks havoc on those who come into the addict's orbit. Because food is so pervasive in our society, it is perhaps the most destructive addiction of all. I went vegan after a moment of clarity when I realized that eating animal products was not just a personal lifestyle choice. It was also a moral choice. I decided that killing and hurting goes against my moral beliefs, not just when it comes to human beings but when it comes to all beings that feel pain and suffering, including cows, pigs, lambs, goats, turkeys, and chickens.

We have a population that has now surpassed the 300 million mark. Think about all those chicken nuggets that people cram into their mouths, pretending they grow on trees. There's a great poster of a beautiful, little yellow chick, and the caption says: "I am not a nugget." Take a guess at how many animals are slaughtered in America for food every year.

Come on, just take a guess (I will tell you the correct answer in a moment).

These animals don't just suffer when they die. Their lives are hellish from the moment of their birth to their last breath. Pigs, which have a higher IQ than dogs, are kept in crates—called gestation crates—just slightly larger than the size of their bodies, never able to turn around or even scratch themselves. It's easier to fatten them up and control them that way. These highly intelligent creatures become psychotic because of the intense confinement. It is simply torture. In fact, according to the brilliant book *Eating Animals* by Jonathan Safran Foer, which I highly recommend, "Every factory-farmed animal is, as a practice, treated in ways that would be illegal if it were a dog or cat."[20] He's absolutely right. If you treated your dog or cat the way cows, pigs, goats, lambs, turkeys, or chickens are routinely treated, you would be arrested.

Americans kill 10 billion animals for food every year. 10 billion! That's a lot of killing . . . a lot of bloodshed, a lot of suffering.

There are very few laws to protect farm animals, even though they have eyes, ears, hearts . . . even though they feel loneliness, pain, and terror. Most Americans love their dogs and cats as members of the family and empathize when they feel pain. Otherwise Americans wouldn't be spending nearly $10 billion a year on veterinarian bills.[21] That's money spent on compassion. But Americans also spend $142 billion per year on cruelty.[22] That's how much beef, chicken, pork, turkey, and lamb we buy. That money is underwriting factory farming. "Don't tell me about farm animals. I don't want to know!" is something I often hear.

Factory farming has been described as an abduction, rape, and murder operation. Baby farm animals are ripped away from their mothers after birth—calves are literally pulled out of the womb and taken immediately away from their distraught mothers. If the "wet" calves are male, they will likely be tethered on a short chain in seclusion until they are slaughtered for veal. The fact that they can't move makes the veal meat more tender. For these male calves, the first steps they will ever take are on the way to their executioner. Female calves enter the madness of dairy farming, where they are artificially impregnated to begin the nightmarish process all over again. The rest are sent to a slaughterhouse to be killed. Abduction, rape, and murder.

We often watch gruesome crime stories on TV, where drug addicts and psychotics do incomprehensible things to other men, women, and children. We gasp in horror and wonder, *How did these people become so evil?* But looking at the violence committed in the name of food, when we eat that food, we need to ask ourselves the same question, *How did we become so deadened to the suffering of other sentient beings?*

> "Our anger, our frustration, our despair, have much to do with our body and the food we eat. The way we eat has much to do with civilization because the choices we make can bring about peace and relieve suffering. When we eat the flesh of an animal with mad cow disease, anger is there in the meat. We are eating anger and therefore we express anger."
>
> —*Thich Nhat Hanh, author of* Anger

In May 2009, talk-show titan Oprah, who is usually a very evolved and sensitive person, offered viewers a coupon for free chicken at a major fast food chain. She announced that the offer for a free, grilled-chicken, two-piece meal would be available for twenty-four hours. By that afternoon, it was the fifth most searched item on Google Trends. Restaurants were mobbed. More than 10 million coupons were downloaded. The chain was thrilled, telling ABCNews.com the reason the company sought out Winfrey to promote the product was "pretty self-explanatory. She's got a huge audience who trust her."[23] Getting the picture? It is heartbreaking to think of the millions of chickens that were slaughtered for that one promotion and alarming to see our nation's meat addiction in full bloom.

Meet the Meat Junkies

Naloxone is a drug used to counter the effects of opioid overdose, for example, heroin or morphine overdose. In the terrific book *Breaking the Food Seduction,* Dr. Neal Barnard writes, "When researchers use the drug naloxone to block opiate receptors in volunteers, meat loses some of its appeal. Researchers in Edinburgh, Scotland, found that blocking meat's opiate effect cut the appetite for ham by 10 percent, knocked out the desire for salami by about 25 percent, and cut tuna consumption by nearly half. They found much the same thing for cheese ... What appears to be happening is that, as meat touches your tongue, opiates are released in the brain, rewarding you—rightly or wrongly—for your calorie-dense food choice and propelling you toward making it a habit."[24] In other words, you can get hooked on meat! Meat and dairy are the staples of fast food—and just as with cigarettes, the business model built on addiction is highly profitable. In the movie *Super Size Me,* the director points out that at least one major fast food company calls its good customers "heavy users."

Americans eat about twice the amount of meat as the global average. We're about 5 percent of the world's population, but we eat more than 15 percent of the meat consumed in the world. Sadly, the rest of the world is starting to imitate us. People in Asia, the Middle East, Latin America, and the Mediterranean, whose diets had been to a great degree plant-based, are now equating meat with affluence and gorging on it too. So they too are developing Western ills, like obesity, heart disease, acne, and diabetes.

In the early 1960s, the world's total meat supply was about 70 million tons. In 2007, it was more than 280 million tons.[25] That's a lot of dead animals. Whether it's a chicken breast on a salad, a slice of bacon on a breakfast sandwich, or the pepperoni on a pizza, each of those animal products came from a living being that cannot exist without those parts. As I always like to say, there's no such thing as "spare" ribs. The average consumer is nibbling on the carcasses of hundreds of animals each year.

It's Destroying the Environment

According to an in-depth United Nations study, meat production is *the single biggest* cause of global warming, far beyond transportation, something even hybrid-driving, liberal Democrats have been trying to ignore, for fear of having to look in the mirror.[26] The wanton destruction of the rainforest is happening primarily to create grazing land for cattle. In one typical five-month period, more than a thousand square miles of Brazilian rainforest were destroyed to create either grazing land for cattle or farmland to raise crops to feed the cattle.[27] Also, consider the methane gas produced by the animals themselves and their mind-boggling physical waste. Think how much excrement 10 billion animals produce (if that doesn't ruin your appetite, I don't know what will). A lot of runoff from factory farms heads down rivers, like the Mississippi, and ends up in large bodies of water, like the Gulf of Mexico, where it's creating aquatic dead zones.[28] Then factor in all the energy expended in growing all the grain, corn, and soy consumed by animals. If you care about world hunger, consider this. If all the "feed" used to fatten up cattle, pigs, goats, sheep, chickens, and turkeys were instead given as food to starving humans around the world . . . we could eliminate world hunger.[29]

In Third World countries, poverty is marked by malnutrition and starvation. In America, poverty is increasingly marked by obesity. The greater Huntington, West Virginia, area was recently designated America's unhealthiest region. The five-county pocket of Americana has a poverty rate of almost 20 percent, which is well above the national average, and about *half* of all the residents are obese! No surprise that the area also led the nation in diabetes and heart disease.[30] Tragically, the dysfunction underlying that region's obesity is becoming the rule, not the exception. Is this really what we want to be?

Given all of these facts, it is obvious that our fast-food lifestyle is simply not sustainable! Now we must ask ourselves, "What can be done?" We can start with more humane farm practices, slashing subsidies to agribusiness, and encouraging consumers to purchase locally grown, organic fruits and vegetables. It's time we stopped endorsing and promoting our own demise.

You Ain't Heavy, You're My Enabler

There's an old saying, "Tell me who you walk with and I will tell you who you are." What that means is you become like the people you spend time with. So, to give yourself a fighting chance against food addiction, hang out with friends who are fit, active, and healthy. You're probably thinking, *You've gotta be kidding, right?* Wrong. A three-decade study of more than 12,000 people published in the *New England Journal of Medicine* showed that a person's chance of becoming overweight rises by 57 percent if he or she has a friend who's overweight, by 40 percent if a sister or brother gets heavy, and by 37 percent if a spouse becomes obese.[31] That likelihood triples among close friends. Study author Dr. Nicholas Christakis of Harvard University called it a "social contagion." It makes sense when you think about it. Associating with overweight people makes being overweight seem normal and acceptable.

Another study, by researchers at the University of Buffalo, found that obese kids consume a lot more calories when they eat with their overweight friends than when they eat with their thin or normal-weight friends.[32] It's easy to say, "Hey, if they're binge-eating on snacks, then it's okay for me to gorge too!" When food addicts get together, the kitchen becomes a drug den. What we should be doing is hanging out with people who challenge and encourage us to be our best selves, not our worst!

In developing food sobriety, it's invaluable to have a social network in place that supports your new, healthier choices. In the vegan world, we call it "vegan kinship." This is a subculture that supports vegetarian choices. We help each other weather the social backlash that comes with going against the tide. It's an enormous comfort to have vegan friends who understand me and with whom I can celebrate compassion.

When We Eat Addictively, We Are Trying to Escape

I've saved the most important aspect of food addiction for last: the emotional component. When discomfort or emotional pain starts to surface, addicts reach for their substance of choice. Druggies go for drugs. Boozers go for booze. And foodies go for food. But in each case, the question we must ask ourselves is the same: What feelings are we trying to escape from?

A book that's become a classic in food-addiction recovery is *Fat Is a Family Affair* by Judi Hollis. She writes, "We are as fat as we are dishonest!"[33] The stuffing of food to create the pleasure rush is about using the brain's opiates to mask emotional pain. The problem with addiction is that once the rush wears off, we're left with the very same emotional problems . . . plus the additional problem addiction brings—in this case, a weight problem. As Dr. Hollis writes, "As long as we keep eating, we can ignore internal messages that say, *Something is wrong here. I'm living the wrong life. I don't belong in this body or these roles.*"

For me, the evidence that I was eating emotionally could be found in the timing of my cravings. When it comes to food, I was always the Night Stalker!

In the mornings when I wake up, the idea of food is actually somewhat nauseating to me. Once I get into work around 12:45 I eat my first meal of the day, usually a healthy mix of salad, veggies, and something soy like tofu or Fakin' Bacon. So far, so good. I remain fairly disciplined until I get off work because I'm so busy I barely have time to eat. Also, I don't really want to eat after they put my makeup on between 2:00 and 3:00 PM, because my face gets smudged (yes, it takes an hour for makeup). Suffice it to say, for most of my day preparing for my show *Issues*, food is not an "issue."

Fast forward to 9:00 PM. I'm home, I'm exhausted, I'm feeling deserving of a treat. And it's at night that I experience free time, which is precisely when suppressed feelings and unresolved issues come to the surface. I'm no longer distracted by work. The uncomfortable feelings are rising up in me and . . . I escape with my most recent drug of choice: food.

It got to the point where I couldn't fall asleep unless I ate something right before I went to bed. Come to find out I was suffering from a common ailment: night eating syndrome (NES)! Here are the symptoms:

- little or no appetite for breakfast
- eating more food after dinner than during the meal
- eating more than half of daily food intake after dinner hour
- recurrent awakenings from sleep requiring eating to fall back asleep

These symptoms fit me to a tee. I was relieved to find an official syndrome that actually explained behavior that felt increasingly out of control and irrational. The last time I experienced a fit of night eating, I finally had the information to do something about it. And it came from *Fat Is a Family Affair*, which brilliantly hones in on which feelings we eat to escape, explaining, "Eating is a substitute for true intimacy and risk. If we want to change our bodies, we have to change our relationships. . . . Problems arise when we try to get nurturance without being vulnerable. The only way to do that is with food. Food is that single, solitary, lonely substance that is ever-ready and never fails. Food never expects anything of us. . . . People aren't quite that predictable or dependable."[33]

Reading that, I realized there was a long-standing personal issue I was too scared to face. Understanding the real dynamic behind my overeating gave me the courage to finally do something about that issue. I ended a relationship that had been weighing me down, literally and figuratively. This freed me up to find a new relationship, which involved taking a risk and having the vulnerability to seek nurturance from another human being, instead of food. Sure enough, the weight started to come off almost immediately and I began returning to normal. To put it in recovery lingo, I was practicing emotional sobriety by finally getting rigorously honest about my real needs and not trying to stuff them.

The Twelve Step approach to healthy, honest eating can be part of a new spiritually based lifestyle. We can get out of our ego-based gluttony and into health and sustainability, for ourselves and the planet. Such a switch isn't about losing weight, but that will happen naturally as we transition to unprocessed, locally grown, organic foods, with an emphasis on fruits and vegetables, nuts and grains. We can turn those beautiful, healthy, environmentally sound choices into a delicious journey.

"What happens in a 12-step meeting is that people's brains are retrained to experience pleasure from different sources. In a 12-step program, it's a group culture that gives those pleasure centers a different source . . . through the camaraderie of the meetings and the celebration of each person's accomplishments. A 12-step meeting, from beginning to end, is designed to give pleasure. The genius of it is they did this before they knew anything about the brain chemistry. The celebration of birthdays, the appreciation of a person with 2 days of abstinence, the appreciation of somebody with 26 years of sobriety—and the hope that there is a system that will help us—is giving pleasure, all the way to the serenity prayer and the hugs at the end. The meetings can give an experience of joy."

—Anne Katherine, author of
How to Make Almost Any Diet Work

Together, we can learn to spot quick diet fixes for what they are: a $40 billion a year rip-off industry. Recovery lingo says: insanity is doing the same thing over and over again and expecting a different result. We've all done the diets. They didn't work. As they say in *Alcoholics Anonymous: Big Book*, "We thought we could find an easier, softer way, but we could not."

A hopeful aspect of one study about diet is that when somebody loses weight, starts eating healthy, exercising, and basically turning their life around, their friends and relatives are more likely to follow suit. You can set the example for your circle of friends and loved ones. It could save your life and theirs.

Chapter Ten
THE SCRUBBERS: Addicted to Cleanliness

Howie Mandel may be the world's reigning germaphobe. The popular comedian, who hosts *Deal or No Deal,* has courageously opened up to his fans about his severe obsession with germs. That signature fist bump he does with contestants on his hit TV show? Turns out it's not just theatrics. It's actually a symptom of his irrational fear of germ contagion. Mandel told ABC News, "In my mind [my hand] is like a petri dish. . . . Otherwise I would spend the day, as I have in the past in my life, in the men's room rubbing and scrubbing and scalding."[1]

Howie Mandel's fixation on organisms so small they're invisible to the human eye has impacted every facet of his life. He shaves his head because it feels "streamlined" and "clean." He refuses to touch money unless it's been washed and shuns handrails and buffet serving trays. He acknowledges having donned surgical scrubs before and after public performances. When he has shaken hands in the past, he admits to having kept hand sanitizer under his desk and obsessively soaking in it. "My hands were raw and I had no antibodies and I started getting warts and it was—I was a mess." It takes guts to share secret compulsions that are clearly embarrassing. I applaud him for his honesty. Mandel says he suffers from obsessive compulsive disorder (OCD). He's one of about 4 million Americans who've been diagnosed with OCD.[2]

But for every clinical case of OCD, legions of consumers are coming down with a behavioral dysfunction that has the appearance of being a not-so-distant cousin. America's 300 million citizens are being fashioned into a zombie army of Stepford Wives and Mister Cleans whose never-ending war against dirt—real or imagined—is not only irrational and self-destructive, it's also killing the planet.

"I'm a clean freak," people often say now with more than a touch of pride. "You could eat off my floor," is another popular refrain. "I can't think unless my house is spotless," is a chant that echoes across the well-manicured cul-de-sacs of suburbia. These people are *bragging* about their fixation on a behavior that's usually a waste of time. At worst, it's a neurotic habit with a host of disturbing repercussions and possible side effects. This trend has, in recent years, turned into a social contagion that approaches the level of mass hysteria.

"We're seeing advertising on TV everyday where women are set up . . . If you are not thoroughly cleaning your house all the time, if you are not running around with a spray cleaner and wiping up the counter after your child, you might just not be a good enough mom."

 —*Erin Switalski, executive director of Women's Voices for the Earth*

Are Clean Freaks Super Freaks?

How did we get this way? Behind every addiction there is a pusher. A drumbeat of TV commercials have—for decades—not so subtly signaled that if we're not using the latest "new and improved" cleaning product, and if our kitchens don't look as gleaming as the sterile ones we see on TV, then we're somehow dirty, smelly, low class, substandard, and inferior. The backstory of how this maddening meticulousness developed begins long before the invention of the television.

The history of America's journey to obsessive cleanliness is a long and tangled one that is brilliantly outlined in Suellen Hoy's book, *Chasing Dirt: The American Pursuit of Cleanliness*. She explains how, in the Mexican-American War (1846–1848), far more American soldiers died of disease than from combat. In the Civil War (1861–1865), dysentery, diarrhea, and disease led to an effort by the Union Army to improve the personal hygiene of soldiers. The emphasis on cleanliness survived the war, having made a lasting impression on many of the soldiers. Cleanliness began making its way into the American psyche. Epidemics of cholera, typhoid, yellow fever, and flu—particularly in cities where the poor lived in filthy, overcrowded conditions—led to cleanliness campaigns in the latter part of the nineteenth century.[3]

European immigration peaked shortly after the turn of the century, and by 1910, more than 13 million immigrants—from Ireland, Italy, and Eastern Europe—were living in America.[4] And, just as is the case today, bigotry greeted these new arrivals. Hoy writes, "Most Americans considered the 'unwashed' to be the millions of immigrants from southern and Eastern Europe who recently arrived in the country's newly plumbed cities. Seeking employment and opportunity they were quickly told that 'Good Health is Wealth,' which could be obtained by keeping clean. . . . Not wishing to appear inferior or recalcitrant, these newcomers tended to agree that 'the American way was the best way.' With few resources and great difficulty, they adopted American habits of hygiene as best they could—not only to stay healthy but also be accepted and 'get ahead.' . . . There was an American way to brush teeth, and an American way to clean fingernails . . . By linking the toothbrush to patriotism, Americanizers clearly demonstrated that becoming American involved a total makeover of personal habits and loyalties."[5] Cleanliness has always been a very loaded subject precisely because it can trigger deep-seated insecurities about one's status in life, insecurities that may trace back generations.

Cleanliness Has Often Been Used as a Code Word

Cleanliness movements often have a subtext. Dirt can become a code word betraying prejudice against the poor, people of color, or people with different cultural values. Is it any coincidence that genocide is often described as "ethnic cleansing"?

By the 1920s, the then-modern American bathroom had become "the shrine of cleanliness." *Chasing Dirt* shows us soap advertisements from that era that cruelly goad eastern and southern European immigrant women into trying to "live up to" American standards despite their "primitive" training.[6]

This association of "cleanliness"—as it's defined by the powers that be—and "class" is still alive and well today, a cultural parasite that can't seem to be wiped out. There's always been a puritanical quality to America's obsession with cleanliness, an *out damn spot* shame over perceived inadequacies in this department that hints this entire subject is about way more than just physical dirt or germs. Showing off one's cleanliness can act as a validation of one's social status. It's a way of saying, "I'm not from the wrong side of the tracks." Advertisers know this and play to that insecurity.

> "If you are a competitor, you certainly cannot win at everything. However, if you have an ability to control something and win, which is 'I will kill the dust bunnies,' it is satisfying. It quiets the voices. I have gained control."
>
> —*Anonymous cleaning addict*

From Cleanliness to Craziness

Addiction is always about excessive behavior. At some point along the hygiene highway, we crossed an invisible border and entered a landscape where sanitation, instead of merely preventing disease, became a *threat* to our bodies and our planet. This line seems to have first been crossed sometime in the early 1900s. Centuries of gritty, strenuous labor were giving way to mechanization and automation. Horses and dusty roads were being replaced by cars and boulevards. It all conspired to make people measurably less dirty than they had been in previous eras. Soap manufacturers, fearing a shrinking market, began inventing new reasons for people to buy their products.

Suddenly Smelling Like Ourselves Became a Cause for Shame

In the book *The Dirt on Clean: An Unsanitized History*, Katherine Ashenburg describes how the soap industry, over the course of several decades, kept raising the bar on cleanliness. In a brilliantly Machiavellian move, corporate America ramped up the definition of "clean" by introducing the notion of . . . BO.

She describes how her mother, who'd emigrated from Germany, "first heard of a newfangled product known as deodorant . . . for 'problem perspiration.'" Ashenburg writes that the shame-based cleanliness campaign intensified over time. "In my generation, standards reached more absurd levels. The idea of a body ready to betray me at any turn filled the magazine ads I pored over in *Seventeen* and in *Mademoiselle* in the late 1950s and '60s. The lovely-looking girls in those pages were regularly baffled by their single state or their failure to get a second date or their general unpopularity, and all because their breath, their hair, their underarms, or—the worst— their private parts were not 'fresh.' . . . There was no way we could ever rest assured that we were clean enough."[7] If that's not a prescription for addictive fastidiousness, I don't know what is. And attitudes toward cleanliness have gotten even more warped in the half a century since those ads appeared.

We're All So Brainwashed, We Can't See How Crazy We're Acting!

One popular instant hand sanitizer on the market today offers ninety-nine reasons to use their product. It's a head-spinning list that includes most physical things we're liable to come in contact with throughout the day including: turnstiles, escalator handrails, handrails of stairs, subway seats and poles, bus seats, gas-pump keypads, car door handles, locks, computer keyboards, the computer mouse, photocopy machine keypads, calculator keypads, staplers, doorknobs, handles, light switches, elevator buttons, office phones, vending-machine keypads, ATM-machine keypads, plastic security buckets at airports, airplane blankets, in-flight magazines, TV remote controls, jump rope handles, weight-machine handles, refrigerator door handles, toys for pets, thermostats, shopping-cart handles, toll-booth tickets, currency and . . . . you get the idea.[8]

Sounds like they would love all their customers to behave as obsessively as Howie Mandel, even though his behavior is classified as a disorder. Are ad campaigns encouraging dysfunctional behavior by trying to paint obsessive cleanliness as normal? It would certainly seem that way.

"We are getting a little nutty as a society with all these germ advertisements . . . On some of the TV commercials, some of the germs have personalities and they look pretty vicious."

—Michael Jenike, M.D., professor of psychiatry at Harvard Medical School

---

An Unnecessary War Against Germs That Really Aren't Our Enemy

Today, commercials for household cleaning products anthropomorphize germs, turning them into ominous cartoon characters with menacing characteristics that are completely out of line with the threat most household microbes actually pose. This is a strategy to encourage people to use stronger, new "antibacterial" cleaning products despite the fact that mere soap, water, vinegar, and baking soda are known to be effective in keeping most household germs at bay.

Why this encouragement? Could it have anything to do with the fact that household cleaning products have become a $30 billion industry, which is continuously developing "new and improved" products to give Americans something more to add to their shopping carts?[9]

American Women Bear the Brunt of Our War on Germs

Women still buy and use most household cleaning products, which is why advertisers focus on them. As one scientist for the organization Women's Voices for the Earth put it, "Companies are working hard to convince consumers, and especially moms, that they need to regularly disinfect every surface in their homes to protect their families from illness, but that's simply not true."[10] An FDA advisory panel has said: *There is no evidence that antibacterial soaps work better than regular soap and water.*[11] None of this would amount to more than a ridiculous, but otherwise harmless, expenditure of money and time except for one thing: the ingredients in these products are not necessarily harmless.

Disinfectant Overkill: How Too Clean May Be Hazardous to Our Health is a report that cites dozens of scientific studies to make a case that there may well be health risks associated with chemicals found in everyday cleaning products.[12]

One antibacterial chemical found in a growing number of household and personal cleaning liquids is triclosan. It was first developed for doctors and nurses as a surgical scrub when somebody got the idea to add it to everyday household cleaners. That kind of reminds me of when Michael Jackson got the bright idea to use a surgical knockout drug called propofol to get some shut-eye at home. Can you say overkill? Tragically, Michael Jackson overdosed and died. While there's no evidence you can experience a lethal overdose by obsessively wiping down your kitchen countertops with triclosan-laced antibacterial products, there are troubling signs that you may be doing yourself more harm than good.

The *Washington Post* reports it obtained a letter the FDA sent to a member of Congress, which said that recent scientific studies raise questions about whether triclosan disrupts the body's endocrine system.[13] Keep in mind the endocrine system involves your glands, which release hormones into your bloodstream. Hormones regulate everything from your mood to your metabolism to your tissue function.[14] The scariest part? The *Washington Post* says triclosan is now found in the urine of three-quarters of our population.[15] And this is just one of several disinfectants over which health concerns have been raised.

Cue the Superbugs

When I was a kid nobody seemed to talk about allergies. Now it seems like every other kid has an allergy or asthma. You'd think we'd be healthier given all those antibacterials we keep using on our hands. But scientists now fear the exact opposite. Germs play an important role in helping our bodies build up their natural defenses. Doctors warn that babies, especially, must be exposed to germs so they can build up the antibodies needed to combat infection. It's called building up a resistance. When we use hand sanitizers, we don't just kill the bad bacteria but also the good germs that have a purpose. Even worse, when bacteria and viruses are constantly exposed to these unnecessarily strong cleansers, antibiotic-resistant germs crop up. They're known as superbugs.[16] Microbiologists fear we are playing Russian roulette with the natural balance of microorganisms.

Being Pretty Is Getting Pretty Scary

For women, the notion of cleanliness is inextricably intertwined with definitions of beauty and sexual attractiveness. In the post–

World War II era, as Rosie the Riveter retired her overalls, American business devised another ingenious way to separate women from their money. On top of preposterous standards of hygiene, they added impossible standards of beauty, developing innumerable cosmetics products to add to the growing list of de rigueur household and personal-cleaning products.

"The reality is that women are still doing about 70 percent of the housework in the average home and that means that they are—by default—being exposed to more chemicals in the home on a daily basis. In addition, we're talking about exposure to chemicals from all sorts of different sources. On average, women tend to use more personal care products per day than men. On average, they use about 15 products per day, which could be exposing yourself to more than 100 different chemicals from those products at a time."

—Erin Switalski, executive director of
Women's Voices for the Earth

There's a growing consensus among environmental watchdogs that female consumers are purposely kept in the dark about the hazards of what they're slathering on their bodies. "Every morning across America, tens of millions of women apply from twelve to twenty 'personal-care' products to themselves, according to the Cosmetic, Toiletry, and Fragrance Association. . . . American women might assume that somebody has been watching to ensure that potential toxins in those ingredients are kept away from intimate contact with the body's largest organ, the skin. They would be wrong."[17] So writes Mark Schapiro in his frightening but riveting book *Exposed: The Toxic Chemistry of Everyday Products and What's at Stake for American Power.* I'm in the news media, and I was shocked to read his claim that "While the cosmetic companies assert that their products are safe, 89 percent of the ingredients used in cosmetics today have not been assessed by either the FDA or by industry."[18] What? We thought they were looking out for us. Now we go into our bathrooms, read the labels on the back of our "beauty products," and wonder, do any of us really know what all those long words mean?

"We don't really know a whole lot about the chemicals that are put into our products. And there is no effective regulatory mechanism for really making sure that the chemicals we are using are safe before they are sold to us in products. We are basically sitting in this world of toxic soup and we have no idea what we are exposing ourselves to."

—Erin Switalski, executive director of
Women's Voices for the Earth

In the mid-1970s, the Toxic Substances Control Act was designed to regulate chemicals. But critics note, in a blanket move, the government grandfathered in about 60,000 chemicals already on the market. Another 20,000 chemicals have reportedly come on the scene since then.[19]

It turns out Americans have a lot more in common with millions of forgotten, suffering laboratory animals than we think. In *The Hundred-Year Lie: How to Protect Yourself from the Chemicals That Are Destroying Your Health*, author Randall Fitzgerald suggests every American has been used—for decades—as a guinea pig in a vast chemistry experiment. He quotes a toxins expert as saying, "The Toxic Substances Control Act of 1976 allows chemicals to be sold and used unless they are proven to be a risk. The EPA, however, does not conduct its own safety tests, but relies on research conducted by manufacturers." Well, what about the FDA? The author suggests, "When it comes to chemicals added to cosmetics and many other personal care products, the FDA knows as much about their safety as you do."[20]

Things have changed only slightly since that assessment. The FDA recently announced it was joining a government effort to predict how chemicals impact human health and the environment called the Tox21 initiative. This effort, led by the Environmental Protection Agency, claims to have screened 2,000 chemicals, with a goal of reviewing 10,000 by the start of 2011.[21] Even so, that would leave tens of thousands of unscreened chemicals in our everyday products. And so far, none of these screenings seems to have resulted in any change to what's for sale on our store shelves.

Why is this such an urgent issue? Estimates are more than 40 billion pounds of chemicals enter American commerce every day![22] And we are absorbing minute quantities of numerous chemicals on a daily basis.

Are We Being Slowly Poisoned?

If we take a massive dose of something, it's relatively easy to tell if your body is having a bad reaction. But when we take in tiny amounts of chemicals on a daily basis, it's harder to figure out if we are hurting ourselves. The chemicals build up over time and can have a cumulative effect. And who knows how all those different chemicals interact with each other within our bodies. The Environmental Working Group notes, "As people apply an average of 126 unique ingredients on their skin daily, these chemicals, whether they seep through the skin, rinse down the drain, or flush down the toilet in human excretions, are causing concerns for human health, and for the impacts they may have to wildlife, rivers, and streams." Just in case you missed it, we apply an average of 126 unique ingredients on our skin . . . every day.[23]

If you think that number is exaggerated, you may want to do a household and grooming products inventory. Count the number of personal cleaning, cosmetics, and household products you pour on your body or come into physical contact with every day. Then add up all the different ingredients in each of those products. You'd likely find that 126 is not such an outlandish number of ingredients after all. Today, most consumer products are filled with a long list of ingredients that, for the vast majority of Americans, are mostly incomprehensible and unpronounceable. My question is: why are we exhibiting such blind faith and assuming that every product we gulp down or pour on ourselves is A-okay for our health when we can't even pronounce what's in all those vials, jars, and bottles?

Is Europe More Advanced Than We are?

The book *Exposed* asks an even more disturbing question: "Is America itself becoming a dumping ground for products forbidden because of their toxic effects in other countries?"[24] The author's argument is that the European Union has taken a leadership role in banning potentially toxic chemicals, with many other countries following the EU's lead, leaving the United States increasingly isolated because of its short-term-profit-over-long-term-cost ethos. When are America's biggest manufacturers going to embrace the reality that nontoxic, environmentally sensitive products won't put them out of business and will protect their customers' health? When we, as consumers, start demanding it!

Sobriety Is About Getting into the Solution

I am definitely *not* an advocate of requiring the government to test all these chemicals by torturing additional millions and millions of laboratory animals to death to determine just how toxic some of them are. We need to simply get rid of a lot of these chemicals! To a large degree, this all boils down to us, *the consumers,* not allowing ourselves to be seduced by manipulative marketing practices and making smarter, more compassionate choices that are in our enlightened self-interest.

For every single chemical-filled product on the market, there is already, today, as we speak, an alternative version without the harsh chemicals on sale at health food stores, cooperatives, Whole Foods, and other environmentally conscious retailers.

From detergents to dish-washing liquid, from toilet cleaner to talcum powder, from shampoos to sunblock, from oven cleaner to underarm deodorants, from lip gloss to eyeliner, you can find products that are cruelty free (meaning they are not tested on animals) and have no artificial colors, flavors, fragrances, or preservatives. Some products even explain the purpose and source of every ingredient on the label. These products are less harmful to the environment, tending to be biodegradable and, obviously, less toxic. If these alternative products can achieve the same results—clean clothes, clean floors, clean dishes, clean mouths, clean hair, pretty lips and eyes—why do we need all those chemicals? The answer is: WE DON'T!

I know those environmentally sensitive products work because I use them. Nobody's accused me of having bad body odor or straw-like hair or a dirty toilet or soiled plates. However, as long as most Americans keep buying the chemical-filled brands, where's the incentive for those manufacturers to change their products? THERE ISN'T ANY!

The List of Chemicals Entering
Our Bodies Just Keeps Growing

The Environmental Working Group did what's called a "body burden" study, testing nine people for more than 200 chemicals. In those nine people, they discovered 167 different industrial and agricultural chemicals, among them: PCBs, dioxins, and insecticide components. Some of the chemicals found have been associated with cancer and birth defects.[25] The interesting thing is most of the test subjects were environmentalists. Even they are overexposed.

We Can't Wait for Government to Act

Let's face it. Thanks to pervasive lobbying and influence peddling, plus a revolving door between government and private industry, our government agencies are, for the most part, controlled by the very companies they're supposed to regulate. It's a morally bankrupt system. Oversight is a joke.

It's time for consumers to take back the power and demand less toxic products. When the economies of scale kick in, alternative products will become as inexpensive as toxic ones. By using the power of our purse, we can all accelerate this trend. In the meantime, it would behoove all of us to examine whether we really need all the different types of products we accumulate in our cabinets and drawers.

Define Cleanliness

The tragic irony is, in our race to be superficially superclean, we have unnecessarily dirtied ourselves with unnatural substances and polluted the world around us. That's the opposite of clean. The more than 40 billion pounds of chemicals that enter American commerce daily have to go somewhere. Ultimately, much of it ends up seeping into the ground water and polluting our rivers and oceans. Is this really the world we want to leave for our children and grandchildren? A world where the lakes, streams, and bays are off limits because they are too dirty to splash in?[26]

"We have no idea what the long-term problems are. All we know is that there is a serious rise in health problems. We are seeing a 40 percent increase in women having trouble getting pregnant in the last 20 years. We don't know why. We have a huge rise in autism. We don't know why. There is a huge rise in learning disabilities. We don't know why."

—Erin Switalski, executive director of
Women's Voices for the Earth

There Is Superficial Clean and There Is Deep Clean

Addictive, ego-based cleanliness is very narrowly focused. It's all about keeping our personal property looking good. We don't leave food to rot on our kitchen counter. We count on the city to pick up our trash each week. Our exacting standards are a source of pride. When people see how "neat" we are, we get a rush of pleasure. That's the addictive hit. We might call this "keeping up with Joneses' cleanliness." What happens to our garbage—once it leaves our property—ceases to be our concern. We turn a blind eye to how our waste might be impacting the environment and wildlife.

Addictive Cleanliness Regards Hygiene as a Zero Sum Game

Either the addict wins or the germs/pests/smells win. It's rooted in fear and manifested by a desire to kill the offending object. Perhaps the most dramatic example of this I've experienced is when a swarm of bees landed on my balcony and some of my neighbors began insisting that I call an exterminator. I went online, did a little research, found that a bee swarm is likely to move on in a couple of days, and I did absolutely nothing and pleaded with my neighbors to be patient. The bees soon left with their lives intact. What a shock. We had managed to coexist. It turns out that honeybee populations are plummeting in what scientists call "colony collapse disorder." Pesticides are among the likely factors.[27] Honeybees are a vital part of our ecosystem as they carry out pollination. Anyway, they're God's creatures. They deserve to live. Besides, when we mindlessly exterminate the "inconvenient" creatures in our midst, we bring dangerous pesticides and chemicals into our lives that can hurt us, our children, and even our companion animals.

Obsessive cleanliness may also be a manifestation of deep-rooted feelings of guilt, shame, and a fear-based need to control our narrowly defined environment in an increasingly frightening and out-of-control universe. I may not be able to exert any influence over this crazy, scary world, but—dammit—I can impose order on my closet.

"Partially it is about control. Control over an intimate, close environment. Control gives me some sort of pay off emotionally."

—Anonymous cleaning addict

Emotionally Sober Cleanliness Is About Letting Go

Emotionally sober cleanliness is about surrendering to life on life's terms, germs and all, and trusting the universe enough to believe that certain tiny creatures—including bugs—were put here by nature for very good reason. If you do find a bug or a spider in your house, why not try your very best to remove it to the outdoors and let it go on its merry way?

When it comes to personal hygiene, emotionally sober cleanliness is an acknowledgment that we are meant to coexist with microbes that are invisible to the human eye and that everything that we encounter by surprise is not our enemy. Emotionally sober cleanliness is about accepting our bodies and trying to keep ourselves clean and pure internally.

A little self-analysis might also help get to the root cause of a cleaning binge. I know when I get the urge to clean unnecessarily, it's often because I'm avoiding something I'm supposed to do, like a writing assignment. Or perhaps I'm trying to "dust away" a resentment. We tell ourselves that by cleaning vigorously, we can rid ourselves of something unwanted. It's like purging. But by throwing it out, are we really getting rid of it? Sobriety is not about dumping something unwanted. It's about processing it.

Garbage, dirt, and waste are never really eliminated. They are only moved from one part of our world to another. Why not embrace the whole world as ours to protect and keep clean? This will inspire us to become concerned about much more than just what happens within the narrow confines of our bathrooms and backyards.

There's a saying in recovery: You can save your face or you can save your ass. One might also say, you can scour your home or you can save the planet.

Chapter Eleven
THE MONGERS: Addicted to War

– – – – – – – – – – – –

There's a reason I've saved the worst for last. While every addict is supremely self-destructive, our nation's addiction to war could—one day—get us all killed. All addiction is progressive. So it stands to reason that our current addiction to war—if allowed to spiral—will invariably lead us into some kind of cataclysmic conflict that could literally wipe millions of people off the face of the earth in a matter of moments. The United States has already proved that one nuclear bomb can destroy a city in a hot second.

The world's first atomic attacks were America's bombings of Hiroshima and Nagasaki some sixty-five years ago. Those two bombs, named Little Boy and Fat Man, turned into massive radioactive fireballs that killed about 200,000 human beings in explosions so violent they literally vaporized people, although many died slow, agonizing deaths from burns and radiation.[1]

Right now, the world has more than 22,000 nuclear warheads, some of which are reportedly thousands of times more powerful than the bombs dropped on Hiroshima and Nagasaki. Thus far, the United States is the only country in history to have used nuclear weapons in warfare.[2] Given that, Americans have a responsibility to take a serious look at whether our modern systems for waging war—and our recent justifications for going to war—have a track record of rationality or whether it's become addictive behavior.

This Is a Patriotic Exercise

We owe it to ourselves—citizens, voters, and taxpayers—and to our children to expose and examine the issue of "war addiction." We have an obligation to America's courageous and well-intentioned soldiers to do due diligence on our rationale for sending them into life-threatening situations. The men and women of our armed forces, who've made so many personal sacrifices to serve our country, should only be asked to risk their lives for an absolutely necessary cause, not a seductive delusion. We can honor our war heroes, maintain the security of our nation, and still examine the addictive component in war. I say this because war addicts, otherwise known as warmongers, are the first to question someone else's patriotism when it conflicts with their grandiose designs for war.

To understand how the concept of addiction applies to our relationship with war, let's revisit how we define addiction. It's an overpowering craving to indulge in a given behavior, followed by bingeing, which is justified through rationalization, followed by remorse, which eventually wears off, allowing the craving to return stronger than ever. Our nation's war cycles fit these criteria. We justified the Vietnam War with the rationalization of the domino theory, binged on war, felt a tremendous remorse, created the antiwar movement, made a commitment to peace, and then—over a few decades—forgot every lesson we learned. It's the same pattern of the drunk who gets arrested, feels remorseful, vows to stay sober, remains sober for a few weeks, and then—when the embarrassment has finally worn off—goes out and gets drunk all over again. Addiction is a disease of amnesia.

"Hopefully it reaches a breaking point where you recognize that you've got a problem. You hit rock bottom where you recognize that you've got a problem . . . you recognize that you've got an addiction and that it is destroying you. And when you finally are willing to come to terms with that, then you do something about it."

—Charles F. "Chic" Dambach, president
and CEO of the Alliance for Peacebuilding

Addictions can rarely be traced to one single cause. I became an alcoholic because of a genetic predisposition (my dad was an alcoholic), environmental exposure (I saw him drink to excess and regarded that as normal), and emotional and psychological reasons (I was using alcohol to check out and suppress childhood traumas). Similarly, there are many factors that lead to our collective war addiction.

The most obvious component is our military-industrial complex. Ironically, while those who bandy the phrase are—today—usually considered lefties, it was Republican President Dwight Eisenhower who coined the term in his farewell address to the nation in 1961, a speech that has served as a haunting prophecy:

"This conjunction of an immense military establishment and a large arms industry is new in the American experience. The total influence—economic, political, even spiritual—is felt in every city, every state house, every office of the federal government. . . . In the councils of government, we must guard against the acquisition of unwarranted influence, whether sought or unsought, by the military-industrial complex. The potential for the disastrous rise of misplaced power exists and will persist."[3]

For the military, the industries that profit from war, and the politicians who are influenced to support war, the stakes are higher than ever. War is getting more and more expensive and, therefore, more and more profitable. By the summer of 2010, the Iraq/Afghanistan wars had cost American taxpayers more than $1 trillion, making those wars, combined, the second costliest conflict in American history, right behind World War II. And that's adjusted for inflation.[4]

If you look at it in terms of cost *per soldier*, Iraq/Afghanistan takes the prize as *the most expensive conflict ever*—even when adjusted for inflation. It cost about $132,000 to house, clothe, equip, transport, and engage a soldier in Vietnam for a year. It costs more than a million dollars a year to keep a soldier fighting in Afghanistan, according to a report in the *New York Times*.[5]

High-tech weapons and aircraft are a big part of the escalating cost. To give you a taste of the money at stake in keeping our war machine at full throttle, there's currently a project in development to make one jet that, with variables, could be used by the Marine Corps, the Navy, and the Air Force. It's called the Joint Strike Fighter plane, also known as the F-35 Lightning II. The military plans to buy almost 2,500 of these planes for about $323 billion dollars![6] This is now on track to become the Pentagon's most expensive weapons project. The main contractor is the nation's largest defense contractor, working in partnership with another defense behemoth. But, as with every addict's grandiose plans, the project has run into trouble. Production costs have reportedly doubled. PBS spoke to defense analyst Winslow Wheeler, who said, "The cost on this thing is out of control, but they're pretending it's affordable . . . We have another five years of, you know, testing and development to go. We have only begun to learn about the problems. And so by the time this thing is done, it will be a record-breaker in terms of nightmares in costs, scheduling, performance."[7]

Just as an exercise, what would all that money buy aside from

2,500 fighter jets? Let's see. Some estimates are $30 billion would provide a year of primary education for every child on earth.[8] Okay, so that still leaves us about $290 billion. Oh, I know. We could end world hunger. The cost of ending world hunger has been price-tagged at about $195 billion a year.[9] So for the cost of over 2,500 fighter jets, we could end world hunger for a year, provide a year of primary education for every child on earth, and still have almost $100 billion left over. Hmmm.

"Our conflict seems to me to be symbiotically tied to our economic system. We need it in order to really create messes that can then be addressed through more production and more consumption. So there is a way in which our lifestyle compels us to be addicted to war."

—Laura Roskos, Ph.D., co-president of U.S. section of the
Women's International League for Peace and Freedom

Did the military contractor get this mind-boggling deal on the strength of its technology alone? Could it have anything to do with this defense contractor having one of the most powerful lobbying arms in Congress? This same contractor is known to spend over a million dollars a month lobbying politicians.[10]

Our military-industrial complex needs war to stay profitable. These bureaucracies have taken on a life of their own and have become self-perpetuating. It helps that war is a fabulous distraction. When we are constantly kept in fear, with multicolored terror alerts, we are too distracted to challenge what our government is doing. Many people are also afraid to speak out for fear of being accused of being unpatriotic.

"The reason why we spend such a significant part of our resources in this country on armaments is because there is a deep fear, and that fear is continually played upon, and we really haven't tapped our own courage to be able to challenge the fear."

−Dennis Kucinich, Congressman (D-OH)
and sponsor of the Department of Peace Act (HR 808)

This is what you might call the macro aspect of our cultural addiction to war. There is also the micro aspect, why war is appealing to certain individuals and groups of individuals. Whatever the drug, we use it addictively if we're using it to escape, stuff painful feelings, or compensate for insecurities. That also applies to war.

War as the Ultimate Expression of Power

From Alexander the Great to Napoleon, history is filled with leaders who physically led their soldiers into battle. Conversely, today, the "leaders" who are the most insistent on the need to send others to their deaths have not experienced any battlefield action themselves. This would describe most of the so-called neoconservatives who were itching to invade Iraq and whose opinions held such sway in the Bush White House after 9/11.[11] Because there's such a clear pattern of hawkish men who've sidestepped military service angling for war, it suggests these men are subconsciously trying to experience vicariously what they'd gone out of their way to miss in practice. In war, as in sex, some fantasies that are degrading when acted out can seem fun when they are simply flights of fancy. What would Sigmund Freud say about these guys and their latent machismo? Could these mongers subconsciously be trying to overcompensate for their sense of inadequacy and guilt in having escaped—thanks to their privileged backgrounds—one of man's most daunting and timeless rites of passage? Are they perhaps telling themselves—in some dark corner of their psyche—*Well, I am doing my manly duty now, by maneuvering us into a war*. Or are they just "getting off" on the ultimate high: power. Are warmongers drunk with power?

In contrast, Dwight Eisenhower, the heroic World War II general who became president, famously said, "I hate war as only a soldier who has lived it can, only as one who has seen its brutality, its futility, its stupidity."[12]

War addiction is not limited to any one party or narrow ideology. The United States has been at war for almost a quarter of its roughly 230-year history, waging war during one out of every five years of its existence.[13] War is no longer an aberration, but something Americans have come to expect.

On the Global Peace Index, which uses a set criteria to evaluate the peacefulness of nations around the world, the United States ranks eighty-fifth among nations, far below our immediate neighbor to the north Canada, which ranks fourteenth and behind the United Kingdom, which is in thirty-first place.[14]

"From a psychodynamic point of view, this is primal. I believe that Freud was right: no matter what people criticize about him. There are two instincts that are primal in humankind: Eros and Thanatos. One is the desire for life, which includes love and procreation and relationship, and the other is the desire for Thanatos, which is aggression and includes war."

—Judy Kuriansky, Ph.D.,
professional therapist, author, and radio host

It has been said that the history of our country is a history of war. Like a recovering alcoholic telling old war stories about his drinking days, we have turned our shared past into a drunkalog, regaling the next generation with stories of past violence. We called World War I *the war to end all wars*. But it didn't. We called Vietnam the *televised war* and predicted watching the gore of it all would inspire us to avoid another one. But it didn't.

With the collapse of the Soviet Union, we are the remaining "superpower," leaving us without a viable enemy. So now we're fighting the "War on Terror," an amorphous war that is all around us, all the time. The War on Terror is an endless war. Despite an unnecessary fiasco in Iraq, we still told ourselves that we needed to continue more of the same in Afghanistan, a country that not so long ago confounded and exasperated the Soviet military. The comparisons to the escalations in Vietnam are painfully obvious.

Here's a Snapshot of Our Addiction to War

It's the image of President Obama getting a Nobel Peace Prize in December 2009, around the very same time he told the nation he was ordering 30,000 more troops into the war zone of Afghanistan.[15] That's the reality of our war culture. A president who got elected as an antiwar candidate still can't resist the siren call of war. Why? Because we, as a culture, are hooked on using war as a solution.

There are those who will dismiss this as a simplistic approach, arguing that war is complex and warning that hasty withdrawals can leave many thousands of innocent civilians dead. But the WikiLeaks release of secret U.S. military documents shows that, during the Iraq war, more than 100,000 Iraqis were killed, 66,000 of them civilians. That was just from 2004 to 2009.[16] With that many civilians dying while we're there, it's hard to argue that we're saving them by prolonging our stay.

One commonality of addictive behavior is constant rationalization and justification. The president explained that we need to get deeper into the war in order to get out! That kind of sounds like, "I need to have a drink in order to get over a hangover."

Addiction creates irrational, wishful thinking. The "get-in-deeper-so-I-can-get-out" strategy is a bizarre and unsound justification for war . . . as was the "domino theory" in Vietnam. But our faith in war is so powerful that it also inspires a very sophisticated and aggressive campaign of justification. Troubled actress/addict Lindsay Lohan offered up tortured explanations of why she missed a crucial court date in Los Angeles while caught partying in France (she claimed she lost her passport) and why her alcohol-monitoring bracelet went off (she claimed someone spilled a drink on her leg). This is what addicts do. They insult our intelligence with outlandish stories delivered with a straight face.

And when it comes to crazy rationalizations, nothing beats an internal Pentagon PowerPoint slide outlining America's war strategy for Afghanistan, which landed on the front page of the *New York Times* in the spring of 2010, a few months after Obama's surge announcement. The bizarre and unintentionally hilarious chart immediately went viral.

Death By PowerPoint

Seriously, the Pentagon PowerPoint slide looks like the overactive doodling of a meth head with a pack of crayons. Military officers call the media sessions that go with illustrations like this "very handy" when the goal is not imparting information. Presentations can be so long and convoluted, reporters are left in a daze. A retired marine

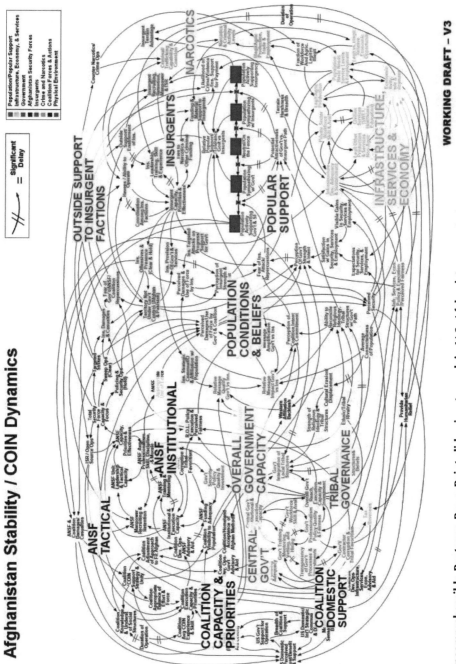

Incomprehensible Pentagon PowerPoint slide aims to explain U.S. Afghanistan war strategy.

colonel calls the process "hypnotizing chickens."[17]

Even the general in charge at that time, Stanley McChrystal, admitted nobody could figure it out. "When we understand that slide we'll have won the war," he remarked dryly.[18]

That same general would soon become a source of derision himself, as the infamous "Runaway General," for offhand remarks he made to a reporter for *Rolling Stone* magazine, which got him fired. General McChrystal and his staff made a slew of derogatory comments about the Obama administration, dismissing President Obama as unprepared for their first meeting and alluding to Vice President Biden as "bite me."[19] That just goes to show you that when you are a full-scale war addict, even 30,000 more troops from a president will not satisfy the craving for more. For an addict, no amount of their drug is ever quite enough. This general's contempt for Obama would seem to stem from his insatiable appetite for war and his intolerance of anybody who might deviate toward a position of moderation, however incrementally. Addicts cannot do moderation. Like we say of drunks, one drink is too many and a thousand isn't enough. Addicts are also reckless and pride themselves on being renegades, which is precisely how this crew of military honchos came off in this behind-the-scenes magazine profile.

Addicts Also Lie Brilliantly

Addicts are so convincing that they often end up believing their own lies. That's because addicts lose touch with the very concept of truth. Their notion of "truth" is whatever enables them to get the result they desperately crave. And usually what works fastest is a lie. This explains how addicts can cajole powerful narcotics out of legitimate doctors. It also explains how America's war-addicted government came up with the faulty information that there were weapons of mass destruction (WMDs) in Iraq, a falsehood that was used to justify our decision to invade a country that had nothing to do with the 9/11 attacks on America.

In his penetrating book *The American Way of War*, author Eugene Jarecki (who also directed the award-winning film *Why We Fight*) lays out how the government has jerry-rigged a system that can manufacture any intelligence result it seeks by cherry picking data. A former Pentagon insider tells him, "There are thirteen different intelligence agencies ... You don't tell 'em what they want to hear, and they will go to other sources ... In the staff meetings we had in the summer of 2002 ... it became clear to me that this war was going to happen. An invasion of Iraq, a toppling of Saddam Hussein, was basically the given. It was just a matter of getting the American people up to speed and getting them behind this effort. Any other means by which Iraq could be dealt with were not discussed."[20]

The author explains that, once a case for war is made, the military-industrial complex kicks into high gear, making massive preparations, which in turn increase the gravitational pull toward war, essentially making it a self-fulfilling prophecy. Does that sound like an addict powerless over the ever-increasing craving to do a drug? It sure does to me. It also reminds us that addiction always leads to moral bankruptcy.

"We know why the people at the top are addicted to war—they profit from it. The bigger question is: why the general public, whose children are being killed and who are going broke financing war, continue to fall for the same fear-mongering parlor trick. Are those people being culturally conditioned to use war for conflict resolution?"

—Blanche DeBeveauville, taxpayer and peace advocate

The-End-Justifies-the-Means Mentality

"The noble lie" elitists use to justify keeping the American public clueless is really not all that different from the crass lie a junkie uses to get his fix. How do the elites get the masses hooked on war? How did they get so many Americans to believe that we had to invade Iraq? Fear. Sobriety is rarely fear based. Addictive behavior almost always is. We were told that we had to take the war to "them" or "they" would take it to us. In truth, what we are really fighting is a state of mind that can crop up anywhere, including Main Street, U.S.A.

On November 5, 2009, my show *Issues* covered the unfolding horror of the worst Muslim-related attack on American soil since 9/11. It did not come from abroad. It was a U.S. Army officer who massacred thirteen Americans and wounded thirty others at our nation's most populous military base, Fort Hood in Texas.[21] U.S. Army Major Nidal Malik Hasan was a devout Muslim psychiatrist who screamed, "Allahu Akbar" (Arabic for "God is great") before he began aiming his gun at men and women in uniform. The *New York Times* noted, "Some experts on terrorism say Major Hasan may be the latest example of an increasingly common type of terrorist, one who has been self-radicalized with the help of the Internet and who wreaks havoc without support from overseas networks and without having to cross a border to reach his target."[22] Of course he's a terrorist. And you are not going to wipe out this brand of terrorism by sending U.S. troops into caves half a world away. In fact, it's believed his upcoming deployment to Afghanistan is what caused this American-born, American-educated lunatic to go over the edge.

It seems every few days there's a new report of a homegrown terrorist. In December 2009, a British citizen was convicted in England of conspiracy to commit murder for his role in a scheme to blow up several transatlantic passenger jets using liquid explosives in the hopes of killing thousands.[23] Sounds like he was trying to pull off a repeat of the 9/11 tragedy, which is precisely what sparked all these wars! But twenty-three-year-old Adam Khatib did not come from the hills of Afghanistan. He was raised in England, attending school in East London before getting a factory job there. Prosecutors say he did ultimately get instruction from foreign militants, but it was on a trip to Pakistan, not Afghanistan. Internet communication also played a key role in this foiled plot.[24] In a global village, with a World Wide Web, terrorism has no borders or boundaries.

> "We made a terrible mistake in even calling this a war on terrorism. Terrorism is a tactic, a way of fighting, the ultimate in A-symmetrical warfare."
>
> *—Charles F. "Chic" Dambach*
> *author of* Exhaust the Limits:
> The Life and Times of a Global Peacebuilder

Addiction Creates Wreckage

The drug addict often destroys his family and imperils his friends. Addiction to war creates a particularly horrific brand of wreckage. More than 5,000 brave American soldiers have been killed in Iraq and Afghanistan. And while the Bush administration often scoffed at the high estimates of Iraqi civilian deaths compiled by activist organizations like Iraq Body Count, it now appears—in light of the WikiLeaks document dump—that the antiwar groups were more on target than our government was willing to admit.[25]

Additionally, the United Nations estimates that, in the first four years of the Iraq war, 4 million Iraqis were displaced from their homes. Some fled the country. Others struggled to survive in impoverished Iraqi shanty towns.[26] How's that for inspiring a resentment against America? What is terrorism, at the end of the day, but a murderous resentment against a more powerful foe and a desire for revenge with religious overtones? Indeed, many theorize that the longer we insist on fighting terrorism with bombs, the more terrorists—homegrown and otherwise—we'll create out of resentment over the resultant carnage.

"We could have had the whole Muslim world on our side if we had continued to do what we started to do. The rest of the world does not like the Taliban or Al-Qaeda . . . at all! But then you go turn on another Muslim country that had nothing whatsoever to do with 9-11? What does that say to the Muslim world? It basically says: We used 9-11 as an excuse to attack Muslims. And that increased terrorism."

—Charles F. "Chic" Dambach, president
and CEO of the Alliance for Peacebuilding

In recovery, we are taught to respect the nameless, faceless people whom addicts tend to mistreat. We are taught not to yell at the anonymous telephone operator, even though we assume we will never meet that person in the flesh. When we, as a culture, disrespect nameless, faceless people on the other side of the world, using the blanket term *terrorism* to justify attacking them, it often comes back to haunt us in the form of still more terrorism. The United States military is now reportedly dropping bombs on selected targets in Yemen, the Arab world's poorest country, which is being touted as "the new Afghanistan" because Al-Qaeda is reportedly establishing a foothold in remote provinces there. There are 23 million people in Yemen. If you kill ten alleged terrorists, there are millions right there ready to take their place. You probably need look no further than at the brothers and cousins of the men killed.[27] Considering every person we kill has numerous relatives, the increase of terrorism is likely to be exponential unless we hit bottom on this obsession with bombing enemies.

In fact, terrorists are starting to use the word *terrorism* against us. The incompetent would-be bomber who, thankfully, failed to blow up an SUV in Times Square in May 2010 told the court, "I am part of the answer to the U.S. terrorizing the Muslim nations and the Muslim people."[28] Faisal Shahzad, while born in Pakistan, was a naturalized U.S. citizen who went to college in Washington, D.C., and Connecticut, ultimately earning an MBA.[29]

One of the key reasons we've yet to hit bottom on our addiction to war is that the average American is so detached from it. It's an abstraction. Surveys show that our wars no longer rank as a high-priority issue among voters. Today, most American citizens are not asked to make personal sacrifices in wartime, like rationing food or gas. America's wealthy and powerful are not likely to see their sons and daughters returning with missing limbs and suicidal thoughts, because America's rich kids almost never go to war. Our all-volunteer military attracts many young people with scant resources and limited opportunities. Yes, the cost of war is sucking up everyone's tax dollars and ballooning our deficits. But on an emotional, physical, and psychological level, it's the common soldier who pays the price.

And What a Price

Suicides and suicide attempts are skyrocketing among American soldiers who've served in Iraq or Afghanistan. In 2007 alone, more than 2,000 U.S. soldiers injured themselves or attempted suicide compared with 350 the year before the war in Iraq was launched.[30] In 2007, more than 120 active-duty soldiers succeeded in killing themselves, the highest level since the army began keeping suicide statistics more than a quarter of a century ago.[31] One in eight returning soldiers are experiencing post-traumatic stress disorder (PTSD), which can include nightmares, flashbacks to traumatic wartime experiences, and other severe emotional and psychological problems.[32]

The enemy's signature weapon, improvised explosive devices (IEDs), which can flip a tank, are creating an epidemic of brain injuries. Beyond the thousands of U.S. troops with penetrating wounds, the *Washington Post* reports "neurologists worry that hundreds of thousands more—at least 30 percent of the troops who've engaged in active combat for four months or longer in Iraq and Afghanistan—are at risk of potentially disabling neurological disorders from the blast waves of IEDs and mortars, all without suffering a scratch."[33]

Romance Versus Reality

Despite this incomprehensible wreckage, we, as a culture, continue to romanticize the drug of war. A drunk romanticizes his alcoholism by remembering the martinis he drank at a stylish bar, not how he ended up puking in the gutter at 3:00 in the morning. Elaborate rituals reinforce the romantic notions surrounding addiction. A cokehead likes his lines on a mirror, a heroin addict has his paraphernalia: the spoon, the needle, and the rope to tie off his arm. A food addict is seduced by colorful candy wrappers.

When it comes to romanticizing an addiction, building rituals around it, and supplying gear for it, nothing tops war. The generals who push for war wear a dizzying array of eye-catching medals, as they talk with each other in obscure, acronym-filled military lingo. It's no accident that President Obama officially announced his troop surge at the West Point Military Academy, in front of hundreds of handsome, fresh-faced cadets who formed a sea of gray at his feet. Steven Spielberg couldn't have devised a more psychologically seductive setting to introduce, to the American people, the very messy subject of escalating a war.

"You can't expect to go somewhere and carpet bomb and expect there not to be ensuing chaos for a long time to come."

—*Matthew Albracht, managing director of the Peace Alliance*

A Pact with the Devil

Another example of war's addictive characteristics: associating with "lesser" companions. Just as a drug addict will end up in the worst part of town hanging out with an unsavory crowd, if that's what it takes to get his fix, so war junkies will partner up with questionable characters in an "ends justifies the means" approach.

Even as President Obama was ordering more troops into Afghanistan, the world was questioning the legitimacy of the Afghan government. Afghanistan's President Karzai was presiding over what is "widely regarded as one of the most corrupt governments in the world," according to the *New York Times*. U.S. generals have described the government as a "crime syndicate."[34] The Afghan president's own brother was "suspected of being a central player in the country's opium trade, a primary source of money for Taliban insurgents," said the *Times*.[35] Wait a second. Aren't those the very people we're fighting?

MAD Stands for Mutually Assured Destruction

Somehow, we still haven't hit bottom on the madness that could land us there. For addicts, withdrawal is very painful. You are deprived of your drug and can feel irritable, sluggish, and even become violently ill. In war, the "withdrawal" is literal but still provokes the same feelings of unease and nausea among those addicted to conflict. One way to get over the pain of withdrawal is to start thinking about starting a new conflict.

Even as we claw our way out of the quicksand of Iraq and Afghanistan, powerful elements within our government are already sounding the drumbeat and making preparations for what could be our next war.

In August 2010, America's highest-ranking military officer disclosed that the United States has a plan to attack Iran. Admiral Mike Mullen, the chairman of the Joint Chiefs of Staff, said, on NBC's *Meet the Press*, "I think the military options have been on the table and remain on the table . . . It's one of the options that the president has. Again, I hope we don't get to that, but it's an important option, and it's one that's well understood."[36]

The justification for what could become America's next war? Same as the last—that all too familiar acronym: WMDs.[37] Admiral Mullen believes Iran's development of a nuclear weapon is an unacceptable risk. Do I believe Iran's claims that it wants nuclear energy simply for peaceful uses? No. Do I think there are ways to deal with Iran's nuclear ambitions that don't have to culminate in bloodshed? Yes. Just like we can create war, we can create peace.

Let's go back to the days after 9/11, when we had a clear choice. We could have gone after the attack's mastermind, Osama bin Laden, with enough determination and resources to catch him and bring him to justice. Then we could have paused to quietly reflect.

Had we done so, we would have realized that we were at a crucial turning point in history. We could have chosen peace.

"America was at a moment where we could have embraced the good will of the world, which was with us in our moment of sorrow, and determined to work with the world community so that nothing like 9/11 would ever happen again. America still needs to embark on a period of truth and reconciliation so that we can set right our moral compass.

"We first have to know the truth, because you can't get to the question of reconciliation or amendment until you know the truth. We don't know the truth because it really hasn't been discussed. There has been no accountability. We are actually living a lie about the nature of the war against Iraq. This is no longer disputable."

—Dennis Kucinich, Congressman (D-OH)
and sponsor of the Department of Peace Act (HR 808)

Making Amends

Many people in recovery from addiction say they made their biggest spiritual leap after admitting their misdeeds and apologizing to those they'd hurt. The process of confession frees an addict from guilt and remorse. It lets us move on in our lives with peace and serenity. It allows us to break through and evolve beyond our self-destructive patterns.

Would our military leaders ever consider doing a formal inventory of the wrongs in the Iraq war, from the faulty WMD intelligence to the Abu Ghraib prison torture scandal and beyond? We all know the story by now.

We need to make amends to those we've harmed. Recovering addicts talk about how they've not only apologized to family and friends but even returned money to employers they've stolen from. Given that we've committed to spending more than $300 billion on 2,500 jets, I think America can come up with peaceful ways to undo some of the damage we've wrought.

Greg Mortenson is the author of *Three Cups of Tea*, which describes how he built dozens of schools in the Taliban's backyard: "The only way we can defeat terrorism is if people in this country where terrorists exist learn to respect and love Americans . . . and if we can respect and love these people here."[38] As part of an amends process, we can easily trade in bomber jets for schools. CARE—a humanitarian organization that fights global poverty—reportedly operates hundreds of schools in Afghanistan, and they've not been attacked by extremists.[39]

If America hits bottom on our addiction to war, we can embark on a journey of emotional sobriety to heal the wounds of war and create alternatives. But we can't wait for our government to do this. The government is broken. It's up to us, individual Americans. Dwight D. Eisenhower saw this movement on the horizon, saying, "I like to believe that people in the long run are going to do more to promote peace than our governments. Indeed, I think that people want peace so much that one of these days governments had better get out of the way and let them have it."[40]

"There really is hard science behind the work of peacebuilding."
—*Matthew Albracht, managing director of the Peace Alliance.*

The Peace Dividend

There is a growing movement among U.S. citizens that is taking a different shape from the antiwar protests of the sixties and seventies. It's called *peacebuilding*. Conflict resolution is a burgeoning field of study in universities. Nongovernmental organizations are joining together to work for peace. In 2009, the first Global Symposium of Peaceful Nations met in Washington, where awards were presented to the world's most peaceful countries.

The financial rewards of nonviolence are being studied as well. The Institute for Economics and Peace says peace on earth would add about $10 trillion to the world economy every year.[41] While some big corporations make billions from war, the vast majority of people lose money and are unable to start new businesses, afraid to travel as tourists, and—of course—there's the tax bills. It's hard to focus on making a buck when you're dodging bullets and mopping up blood.

"Conflict is inevitable. Violence is not."

—Matthew Albracht, managing
director of the Peace Alliance

So what is the secret to peacebuilding? Charles Dambach's biography *Exhaust the Limits: The Life and Times of a Global Peacebuilder* lists the keys:

- Always be on the side of peace
- Listen, really listen to learn and understand
- Demonstrate respect
- Build trust
- Be patient and
- Be persistent[42]

I would add one additional key: **imagine peace.**

"We've lost our capacity to imagine an alternative to war. We need to regain that capacity. We need to understand that peace is not simply the absence of war; it's the capacity for renewal, for transformation, for growth, for benign social and political discourse. We have to re-imagine our democracy as including this potential for peace which, frankly, was there at the founding."

—Dennis Kucinich, Congressman (D-OH)
and sponsor of the Department of Peace Act (HR 808)

It's difficult to imagine a world without war. But a couple of hundred years ago, it was impossible for most Americans to imagine a world without slavery. Eventually people made the evolutionary leap. So it's conceivable that we could also end war. But the first step is to open our minds and imagine the possibility. Buddhist philosopher Thich Nhat Hanh sums it up in his book *Peace Is Every Step*, writing, "Peace is present right here and now, in ourselves and in everything we do and see. The question is whether or not we are in touch with it."

Chapter Twelve
THE SOBERS: Emotional Sobriety

We look back on medieval times and marvel that women were actually forced to wear chastity belts. We gasp as we read about ritualized human sacrifice by the Aztecs. We shake our heads when we think about the Salem witch trials or America's slave trade. We find it hard to believe that American women only won the right to vote in 1920. We look back at segregation and wonder how so many people could have blindly accepted sick manifestations of prejudice. It's only in hindsight that a culture's irrationality, absurdity, and cruelty become obvious to everyone. When we're in the thick of it, grappling with daily issues, it can be hard to see the big picture objectively. When we're brought up to accept something as normal, it can be difficult to condemn and reject it, even when it's diminishing us.

Today, in America, slavery is alive and well. You are a slave and so am I. Our shackles are invisible but strong. Today, slavery is a state of mind, a twisted belief instilled in our psyche that says we can consume, indulge, and bully our way to happiness and success. It's a form of mob psychosis. What we think is normal is really nuts.

We think our drug is the solution when it's actually the problem.

We drink alcoholically to get relief from the strain of life, unable to recognize that boozing increases the stress of life.

We pop prescription pills to alleviate our anxiety and, in short order, pill popping causes even bigger problems than the ones about which we were originally anxious.

We eat over our emotional issues, ignoring the obvious fact that life's inevitable struggles and humiliations are only compounded when we are walking around with pounds and pounds of extra weight.

We buy lots of stuff we don't need to feel more secure about our place in the world, blind to the truth that all these possessions quickly become new responsibilities that drag us down and drain us financially.

We gorge on violent entertainment in the hope of distracting ourselves from our mundane existences, only to feel queasy and nervous, even double-checking our doors, after watching hours and hours of back-to-back murders.

We waste our time and energy obsessing over celebrities we'll never meet in the irrational hope that somehow their glamour and charisma will rub off on us.

We keep our heads buried in high-tech toys as a miraculous world passes us by.

We buy a slew of chemical-laced cleansers and beauty products, telling ourselves this is what we need to be really clean and pretty, when—in fact—it's those very products that are making our world dirty and ugly.

We send our brave American soldiers to foreign lands on ill-defined missions and watch them die and get maimed, physically and psychologically, as our amorphous enemy uses our missteps as a recruiting tool.

And, like every addict, we keep doing it over and over again and expecting a different result, hoping somehow that, on the next try, we'll finally get it right. The wanting never ends. The glory of one acquisition or engorgement quickly fades into disillusionment, leading to a craving for the next. This is the cycle of addiction.

Faux Freedom

We tell ourselves we are making these choices of our own volition. But, in truth, these choices are being made for us. An addict is precisely the person who lacks the power to say no. An addict is, by definition, the person who is powerless in the face of temptation. You get a craving to eat or shop or pop, and you grapple with the urge for a few seconds but ultimately succumb and indulge. You are not making a free choice. You are an addict giving in to the inevitable. The same reasoning applies to groups of addicts.

As an Addict Nation, we are letting others write our life stories for us. The media, corporations, and government bombard us with images and messages about how we should live, what we should wear, what we should eat, who we should have sex with, and who we should consider our enemy. These powerful forces like to script our behavior for their own self-interest, not ours. But the script they've written is at worse a tragedy, at best a farce.

Addicts Live in a Paint-by-Numbers Universe

Powerful interests draw the outlines of our lives and then convince us that freedom is being allowed to choose the color paint we want to use to fill in the blanks. By moving in uncritical lockstep with narrow social norms, we are robbing ourselves of our uniqueness. No two human beings look exactly alike. No two human beings should try to live exactly alike. But we do. From childhood on, we yearn to conform so we can be accepted and liked. It doesn't work. It usually just makes us miserable. The people who are most charismatic are those who break the mold and allow themselves to be what nature intended: an original.

It's time we each start writing our own stories. America became a world power because of rugged individualism, not blind conformity. Freedom from cultural addiction means personal liberation: mentally, emotionally, physically, and financially. It means being your own person.

A Moment of Clarity

So how do we break through and kick these socially accepted forms of self-destruction? First, we must experience a moment of clarity. We have to take an objective look at our behaviors, and instead of asking if other people think it's okay, ask ourselves, *Does this really feel right? Is this environmentally sound? Is it financially sound?* And the most important questions, *Is this morally right? Is my behavior ethical?*

Often, an honest answer to those questions will take some investigation. The worst cruelties on earth are kept hidden far, far away from those co-conspirators we call consumers who want—more than anything—deniability. We would rather not think about the big picture if it's disturbing or distasteful and conflicts with the concept we have of ourselves as "a good person." But in the words of Albert Schweitzer, "No one must shut his eyes and regard as nonexistent the sufferings of which he spares himself the sight."

Do we consumers have the courage to learn about the factory farm that produces our eggs? Will we take into consideration the working conditions of the sweatshop that makes our shirts? Or look into the business practices of the companies we buy stock in? Are we willing to look up the chemicals listed on the back of our shampoo, deodorant, and laundry detergent? And if we find ourselves ethically opposed to what these corporations and brands are up to, will we finally make more sober choices?

Admitting a Problem Is the First Step

What we need to develop, more than anything else, is self-awareness. After all, what is a "habit" anyway but something that we do by rote, almost unconsciously. So to break a bad habit, or a dozen of them, we must first become conscious. Every day we all make hundreds of decisions. We must learn to slow down enough so that we can observe ourselves in the process of making those choices. Then we can learn to stop ourselves before we take an action reactively, reflexively, and unthinkingly.

Whether it's watching a violent movie, eating an unhealthy fast food meal, or blindly marching to the drumbeat of war, we can learn to first ask ourselves, *What are the repercussions of this decision? How is this choice going to impact me and the world around me? What is my responsibility to myself and to this earth? Are lazy, shortsighted choices making my life unmanageable?* We must take off our blinders and get honest about how our cultural addictions are hurting others and the planet.

The Happiness Test

One way to encourage change is to acknowledge that our addictive consumptions are not making us any happier. While those whose basic needs and comforts are met report greater levels of happiness than those who are struggling to survive, there is no correlation between excessive, addictive consumption and happiness. Quite the contrary. Americans—the biggest consumers on the planet—are not the happiest, most content people on earth, according to numerous surveys. In a Gallup World Poll, the United States came in at number sixteen for overall well-being and number twenty-six for enjoyment.[1] Think of that the next time you reach out to make an unnecessary purchase.

Once we have that *aha* moment and avoid a toxic choice, we can then take the next step and move toward a more evolved alternative. One thing we know about addiction is that you can't just take away an addict's drug and leave it at that. You have to substitute it with something that is ultimately more rewarding. It's a trade up. This new "something" may not give you a rush or an immediate high because it's a different kind of pleasure. Sobriety offers a more incremental, more subtle payoff. But it's one that is ultimately much more powerful, fulfilling, and enduring.

Defining Sobriety

Since this is an intervention for an addicted nation, the goal—obviously—is to reach to the polar opposite of addiction. That is called sobriety. So what exactly is sobriety? With alcohol and drugs, you can define sobriety as the state of being 100 percent free of mood-altering substances . . . period. It's that simple. That's a literal definition of sobriety. But for many of the behavioral addictions covered in this book, a broader concept of sobriety is required. That's why recovery work also focuses on "emotional sobriety."

I would define emotional sobriety as being comfortable in your own skin, living in the present moment, facing life with courage, grace, kindness, compassion, humility, and humor, avoiding the temptation of self-destructive escapism, being about something more than yourself, and caring about others and the greater world while taking care of your own needs.

Let me say for the record, there are many, many times when I am not emotionally sober. When I fall off the spiritual beam, for whatever reason, I immediately begin regressing to my old alcoholic personality. I become irritable and discontent and quickly start to develop resentments, grudges, and a victim mentality. I get a chip on my shoulder. I become unpleasant to be around and am prone to yelling. In short, I go negative.

A recovering addict, whatever drug they've given up, is always moving in one direction or the other, either toward more emotional sobriety or away from it and toward a relapse. As a recovering alcoholic, I can't sit back and say, "Well, I've been sober more than fifteen years. I no longer have to work on my recovery." That's a disaster in the making. When I stop working on my spiritual condition, in very short order, the "ism" of alcoholism comes right back, even though I'm not drinking alcohol. They say the "slip" back into the disease happens long before that first drink is picked up. So, perhaps most of all, emotional sobriety is a joyful attitude toward life.

Addiction Is a Disease of the Mind

How do we achieve this "attitude adjustment" that takes us from addictive thinking to emotional sobriety? The seeds that sprout a sober disposition are perfectly outlined in the Twelve Steps of recovery. Based on timeless spiritual principles, the Twelve Steps were first outlined in Alcoholics Anonymous, originally published in 1939. Those same Twelve Steps are now used by millions of people across the globe seeking a reprieve from a plethora of addictions.

The beauty of the Twelve Steps is that it's a very simple set of recovery principles that can be applied to every addiction imaginable, including prescription and illegal drugs, food, sex, technology, materialism, cleanliness, violence, incarceration, celebrity, procreation, and war. They call recovery a simple program for complicated people. Given the complex nature of the addictions covered in this book, perhaps we can amend that to say recovery offers a simple program to deal with complicated addictions.

To make it even simpler, these recovery steps can be reduced to a mere handful of concepts that can guide us through whatever addictive challenge and psychological-emotional issue we encounter.

The simple concepts are:

- surrendering to the truth that we are powerless over our addictive cravings
- recognizing that ours is a spiritual problem with a spiritual solution
- seeking guidance from a higher power as we define it
- writing a list of the damage we've done
- admitting to another person what we've done wrong
- making amends to those we've hurt
- being of service to others

There is an emotional alchemy that occurs when people practice the recovery principles of honesty, humility, integrity, service, and surrender. There is a radiance to someone who is emotionally sober, which is palpable. I recognized that rare quality in a woman who became my first mentor in sobriety fifteen years ago. We've been friends ever since. She's always impeccably dressed, with a refined bearing. But when she starts talking, she's shockingly honest about herself. She laughs as she tells embarrassing stories about her drinking days. She also isn't afraid to share the pain she has experienced. She's humble, especially when it comes to describing how she hit bottom on booze and then turned her life around, trading in her jaded lifestyle for a more spiritual approach. She spends a lot of time helping people like me maintain their sobriety. She's very patient, but also firm and able to set boundaries. In this, and other ways, she is always being of service to others. I would describe this friend as sober, both in a literal and an emotional sense. Her life is in balance.

In an Addict Nation that constantly tells us "You can have one more," it's difficult to know when you've crossed the line into a self-destructive, addictive pattern. If we're overweight, if we're deeply in debt, if we're overworked or frequently tired, if we've got an ulcer or high cholesterol—these are all indicators of a life out of balance. Doing an "inventory" can help us see clearly where we're off track. By keeping a running catalogue of our actions, by literally writing down every cent we spend or every calorie we eat, or everything we drink, or every curse word we use, or every time we lie, or how many products we pour on our bodies, or how many shoes we own, or how many times we text, we can inventory our behavior and get a crystal-clear picture of what's askew. The writing on the page will tell a story we cannot rationalize away. It stares us in the face, and we can no longer say, "It's not that bad." If you're struggling with overconsumption, do a consumption inventory and list every single thing you purchase or use. After a week you may well hit bottom on overconsumption.

Addictions Are Contagious

One thing we know about addiction is that somebody else's bad habits can easily rub off on you. People have a tendency to do drugs in groups, get drunk in groups, and get fat in groups. We've discussed that people are more likely to become overweight if they have overweight friends. There's a recovery phrase for friends who are more severely addicted than you are: *lesser companions.* If you want emotional sobriety, then avoid people who consume addictively and seek out people who have qualities to which you aspire. The same concept applies to places. If you're trying to reduce your consumption, don't frequent superstores, malls, and outlets. Individual decisions, added together, are the only way our culture is going to evolve.

The miracle of recovery is one addict listening to another and identifying with the other person's experience. When two or more people with the same problem connect, there is no passing of judgment or assigning of blame since everyone is in the same predicament. There are recovery meetings, support groups, clubs, organizations, and less formal gatherings for almost every human addiction and predilection. If you've kicked fast food by going vegan, it helps to make friends with other vegans and become part of that healthy, compassionate community. If you're antiwar, it's useful to join an organization that promotes peace . . . and there are hundreds of choices just a Google search away. If you're kicking harsh chemicals and buying organic, you might want to join a health food cooperative where you're likely to run into other ethical shoppers who share your beliefs. It doesn't have to be you against the world. A sense of community and belonging is especially crucial when you've chosen a less-traveled road.

A great example of this is the 100 Thing Challenge. A San Diego father of three named Dave Bruno decided he wanted to "break free from the confining habits of American-style consumerism." So he challenged himself to reduce his material possessions to 100 things, with reasonable exceptions for shared family items.[2] His challenge took off, and now a whole bunch of people are trying the same thing. They've got a Facebook fan page and are developing a community.

Be the Change You Want to See in the World

The Internet is democratizing change. Anybody with a fresh idea can now create a community online. The only way we are going to change our addict-centric institutions is if we join together and invent alternatives. No longer do we have the excuse that it's useless to try because one person alone can't make a difference. We have now truly become a global village where no one has to do it alone.

As you change, you're likely to see everything around you change:

your friends, your belongings, your social life, your goals, and your dreams. As they say of sobriety, the only thing that has to change is . . . everything.

Once an addictive behavior is given up, the recovering addict must always be alert to protect and guard their sobriety. The goal is to achieve and maintain constant serenity. This can be done by avoiding the state of HALT, something recovery programs recognize as a fast track to failure. HALT stands for Hungry-Angry-Lonely-Tired. If you are all of these—at once—you are likely to feel destabilized and your emotional sobriety is bound to dissolve to be replaced with anxiety, stress, resentment, and exhaustion. Eating right, sleeping enough, working through resentments by acknowledging your part in them, and avoiding isolation by making meaningful connections with other evolved people—these are the foundations of a balanced life.

Beyond Ego and Fear

The most crucial component of emotional sobriety is the surrender of ego and the acceptance and strengthening of what some people like to call God consciousness. The ego has always existed. Our ancestral cousins, the apes, display ego. And so do we. The problem is that we modern humans now have so many ways to indulge, bolster, and display our ego that the manifestations of our narcissism are threatening to destroy our physical world. From the big ticket items—houses, cars, boats—to the never-ending supply of disposable trinkets, toys, and conveniences (and everything they come wrapped in), we are now in danger of literally drowning in the debris of our insatiable desires.

In *A New Earth: Awakening to Your Life's Purpose,* Eckhart Tolle brilliantly explains why we've become addicted to consumption, which he calls an insatiable hunger. *"Having*—the concept of ownership—is a fiction created by the ego to give itself solidity and permanency and make itself stand out, make itself special . . . No ego can last for long without the need for more. Therefore, wanting keeps the ego alive much more than having . . . And so the shallow satisfaction of having is always replaced by more wanting. This is the psychological need for more, that is to say, more things to identify with. It is an addictive need, not an authentic one."[3]

It stands to reason that, when you finally know who you are and feel that you *are* enough, you will no longer need to use *things* to solidify your identity and you will feel that you *have* enough.

I wrestle with my ego as much, or more, than the next person. There's a reason I've been on television for most of my life. I like to be seen and I like to hear myself talk. Here's a confession: when I'm alone, I often talk to myself. To my great embarrassment, I've been overheard giving speeches in the bathroom.

EGO: Edging God Out

I also struggle with overconsumption and, like most consumers, find myself lusting after shiny objects. But the other day, I had what I consider a breakthrough. I saw a beautiful luxury car on the street. It was painted an enticing baby blue and just glimmered. My first thought was, *Oh, I'd love to have that car.* But then I caught myself and wondered, *Why did I just have the urge to possess the car, as opposed to just appreciating its beauty in and of itself?* After all, I live in Manhattan and don't even need a car. Ego, of course. My ego desired to devour that car and make it part of my identity to bolster my sense of self. Some reptilian part of my mind calculated: Jane plus nice car is better than just Jane. But then I said, "No, that's not true. The shiny, blue car is not going to make me any better."

The moment I had this realization I suddenly became aware of another part of me that felt larger than my ego-based identity. It was as if I was invisible and melded into the sky, observing the visible Jane down on the street. This larger part of me decided to just stare at the car and appreciate its sleek design and polished chrome and try to let go of my ego's desire to own it. For a few moments, I felt freedom from what I would call "little Jane" and felt the presence of "big Jane." And then a dichotomy emerged. I got this marvelous feeling that the entire world was mine and everything in it belonged to me. Therefore, there was no need to technically "own" anything that I didn't genuinely need. Put another way, I recognized within myself what you could call God consciousness. God consciousness is very hard to hold on to, but I keep trying. It's like free falling, exhilarating once you get over your fear.

A Life of Service

So what's the ultimate alternative to an egocentric/addict-centric life? When we finally get the meaninglessness of endless acquisition, when we finally understand the tired cliché "You can't take it with you," then we look around and say, "Well, now what am I going to do with my money, my time, and my energy?" Thankfully, there are millions of things that need doing. You don't have to become a full-fledged activist to have a life of purpose. You can simply be of service to another person or creature in need. You can visit an isolated senior citizen, foster a neglected child, or exercise the dogs at the local shelter. Tithing a set portion of your income is an admirable way to purposefully direct those disposable dollars that used to go into a gaudy decoration or another outfit you don't really need. For the cost of a cheap suit, you can enable doctors with Smile Train to repair a child's disfiguring cleft lip and change someone's life forever.

What would our society look like if we all became willing to transcend our materialistic values? What would our culture look like if we all evolved beyond our most hideous ego-based compulsions? It would be a completely transformed society: less focused on pride and fear and more focused on self-knowledge and caring for each other. It would be a society less interested in hate and war and more interested in love and peace, a society less inclined to ugliness and more to beauty. It would be a world less focused on punishment and more adept at preventing crime. It would be a culture with more "matriarchal" values, like compassion, protection, forgiveness, and unconditional love. We'd all enjoy a much more serene lifestyle.

Addiction brings out the worst in us. When we finally give it up, we experience a new, natural high as we're freed from the bondage of craving. Some call it a fourth dimension.

Together, we can evolve. The promise of cultural sobriety is a safer, more peaceful America that will give all of us a better shot at the pursuit of happiness.

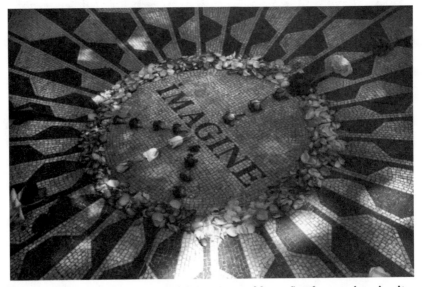

Before we can achieve a peaceful, joyous world, we first have to imagine it.

ENDNOTES & INTERVIEWS

Introduction

1 "Bet You Can't Eat Just One," *The Atlantic*, March 29, 2010, http://www.theatlantic.com/ food/archive/2010/03/bet-you-cant-eat-just-one/38181/.

2 See "1,000,000,000 Live in Chronic Hunger and I'm Mad as Hell," Food and Agriculture Organization of the United Nations, http://www.fao.org.

3 On war profiteering, see "The SIPRI Top 100 arms-producing companies, 2008," Sipri.org., http://www.sipri.org/research/armaments/production/Top100; "Top 100 Defense Contractors," GovernmentExecutive.com, August 15, 2007, http://www. govexec.com/features/0807-15/0807-15s3s1.htm; and Adam Levine, "Halliburton, KBR sued for alleged ill effects of 'burn pits,'" CNN, April 28, 2009, http://www.cnn.com/ 2009/US/04/28/burn.pits/index.html.

Chapter 1: The Stuffers

1 Robert Frank, "Millionaire Says Money 'Prevents Happiness,'" *Wall Street Journal*, February 9, 2010, http://blogs.wsj.com/wealth/2010/02/09/millionaire-says-money-prevents-happiness/.

2 Eviana Hartman, "Wrapping Paper: Using It Is Bad, Burning It Is Worse," *Washington Post*, November 23, 2008, http://www.washingtonpost.com/wp-dyn/content/article/2008/11/20/ AR2008112003358.html; and Waste Facts and Figures, Clean Air Council, http://www.cleanair.org/ Waste/wasteFacts.html.

3 "Tops in 2008: Most Popular Consumer Goods," NielsenWire, December 18, 2008, http://blog.nielsen.com/nielsenwire/consumer/tops-in-2008-most-popular-consumer-goods.

4 Packaging on Seventh Generation brown paper towels, accessed on Facebook, http://www.facebook.com/group.php?gid=16518050343.

5 Amy Cassara, "Ask EarthTrends: How Much of the World's Resource Consumption Occurs in Rich Countries?" blog entry, World Resources Institute: EarthTrends, August 31, 2007, http://earthtrends.wri.org/updates/node/236.

6 Nancy Gibbs, "One Day in America," *Time*, November 15, 2007, http://www.time.com/ time/specials/2007/article/0,28804,1674995_1683300,00.html.

7 Anxiety Disorders Center: Compulsive Hoarding, Hartford Hospital, http://www.harthosp. org/InstituteOfLiving/AnxietyDisordersCenter/CompulsiveHoarding/default.aspx#QA.

8 See *Hoarders* on A&E TV (http://www.aetv.com/hoarders/about/) and *Hoarding: Buried Alive*, on TLC network (http://tlc.discovery.com/tv/hoarding-buried-alive/).

9 Oskar Garcia, "Body of Las Vegas woman found in clutter at home," *Associated Press*, August 27, 2010, http://www.fox12idaho.com/Global/story.asp?s=13055966&clienttype= printable.

10 Bureau of Economic Analysis National Economic Accounts, U.S. Department of Commerce, June 2010, http://www.bea.gov/newsreleases/national/pi/pinewsrelease.htm.

11 Louise Story, "Home Equity Frenzy Was a Bank Ad Come True," *New York Times*, August 14, 2008, http://www.nytimes.com/2008/08/15/business/15sell.html?_r=1.

12 Ellen Bowman, "Where All the Retirees Are Above Average," The Motley Fool, http://www.fool.com/personal-finance/retirement/2007/04/19/where-all-the-retirees-are-above-average.aspx.

13 Martin Lindstrom, *Buy•ology: The Truth and Lies about Why We Buy* (New York: Crown Business, 2010), 20.

14 Ibid., back cover.

15 Ibid., 11.

16 Ibid., 32.

17 Anup Shah, "Poverty Facts and Stats," Global Issues, March 28, 2010 (updated September 20, 2010), http://www.globalissues.org/article/26/poverty-facts-and-stats.

18 Paco Underhill, *Why We Buy: The Science of Shopping: Updated and Revised for the Internet, the Global Consumer, and Beyond* (New York: Simon and Schuster, 2008), 24.

19 Ibid.

20 Enoughism.org, http://www.enoughism.org/; and see "enoughism," Wikipedia, http://en.wikipedia.org/wiki/Enoughism.

21 Sloan, "What's Still Wrong with Wall Street," *Time*, November 9, 2009.

22 Intentionally omitted.

23 Annie Leonard, *The Story of Stuff: How Our Obsession with Stuff Is Trashing the Planet, Our Communities, and Our Health—and a Vision for Change* (New York: Free Press, 2010), 99.

24 Ian Urbina, "BP Used Riskier Method to Seal Well Before Blast," *New York Times*, May 26, 2010, http://www.nytimes.com/2010/05/27/us/27rig.html.

25 CNN Wire Staff, "Oil inspectors took company gifts, watchdog group finds," CNN online (U.S. edition), May 25, 2010, http://www.cnn.com/2010/US/05/25/oil.spill.interior/index.html.

26 Charlie Savage, "Sex, Drug Use and Graft Cited in Interior Department," *New York Times*, September 10, 2008, http://topics.nytimes.com/topics/reference/timestopics/people/s/charlie_savage/index.html, accessed May 25, 2010.

27 "Everyday Uses of Oil," Paleontological Research Institution, http://www.priweb.org/ed/pgws/uses/plastic.html.

28 Brian Handwerk, "Giant Ocean-Trash Vortex Attracts Explorers," *National Geographic* online, July 31, 2009, http://news.nationalgeographic.com/news/2009/07/090731-ocean-trash-pacific.html.

29 Tim Jackson, *Prosperity Without Growth: Economics for a Finite Planet* (London: Earthscan Publications, 2009), 184.

30 Anup Shah, "Poverty Facts and Stats," Global Issues, March 28, 2010 (updated September 20, 2010), http://www.globalissues.org/article/26/poverty-facts-and-stats.

Chapter 2: The Pharmers

1 Natalie Finn, Ashley Fultz, and Lindsay Miller, "Michael Jackson's Parents Fume, Say Conrad Murray 'Killed Him,'" E Online, February 8, 2010, http://www.eonline.com/uberblog/b166241_michael_jacksons_parents_fume_say.html.

2 "The Drugs That Caused Michael Jackson's Death," Reuters, February 8, 2010, http://www.reuters.com/article/idUSTRE6174A420100209.

3 "Jacko Sued for Not Paying for His Meds," TMZ, January 12, 2007, http://www.tmz.com/2007/01/12/jacko-sued-for-not-paying-for-his-meds/.

4 "Geller, Ex-bodyguard Tell of Jackson Drug Abuse," Associated Press, July 2, 2009, http://today.msnbc.msn.com/id/31706977; and Paul Solomon, "Opinion: Did Prescription Drugs Kill Michael Jackson?" *Digital Journal*, July 2, 2009, http://www.digitaljournal.com/article/275152.

5 Karlie Pouliot, "Drugs That Killed Heath Ledger Could Be in Your Home," February 6, 2008, Fox News.com, http://www.foxnews.com/story/0,2933,328926,00.html.

6 "Anna Nicole Smith died of accidental overdose," Associated Press, March 27, 2007, http://www.msnbc.msn.com/id/17788386/page/2/print/1/displaymode/1098/.

7 "Arrest Linked to Corey Haim Death," CBS/Associated Press, March 13, 2010, http://www.cbsnews.com/stories/2010/03/17/entertainment/main6308582.shtml; and Mike Fitgerald, "Hillbilly Heroin: The Story of Jon Riley Hays, M.D.," Opiates.com, *Belleview News-Democrat*, http://www.opiates.com/media/heroin-belleville.html.

8 Lisa Fletcher and Sarah Netter, "Corey Haim: Where Did His Prescriptions Come From?" ABC News.com, March 15, 2010, http://abcnews.go.com/GMA/corey-haim-death-prescription-drugs/story?id=10099842.

9 Nancy Dillon, "Corey Haim autopsy results: Former child actor died of natural causes, not a drug overdose," *New York Daily News*, May 4, 2010, http://www.nydailynews.com/gossip/2010/05/04/2010-05-04_corey_haim_autopsy_results_reveal_actor_died_of_natural_causes_not_a_drug_overdo.html; Robert Jablon, "Corey Haim Cause of Death: Pneumonia Complications, NOT Drugs," Associated Press and *Huffington Post*, May 4, 2010, http://www.huffingtonpost.com/2010/05/04/corey-haim-cause-of-death_n_563300.html.

10 Liz Szabo, "Prescriptions now biggest cause of fatal drug overdoses," *USA Today*, October 2, 2009, http://www.usatoday.com/news/health/2009-09-30-drugoverdose_N.htm.

11 Barry Meier, "When Pain Drugs Hurt: Focusing on Doctors," *New York Times*, CNBC online, July 29, 2010, http://www.cnbc.com/id/38464522.

12 California Office of the Attorney General, Cures Program, http://ag.ca.gov/bne/cures.php.

13 National Drug Control Strategy FY 2009 Budget Summary, White House, February 2008, http://www.cfr.org/publication/10373/forgotten_drug_war.html; http://articles.cnn.com/2009-03-31/politics/cafferty.legal.drugs_1_drug-trials-cartels-drug-suppliers?_s=PM:POLITICS; http://www.whitehousedrugpolicy.gov/publications/policy/09budget/index.html.

14 Liz Szabo, "Prescriptions now biggest cause of fatal drug overdoses," *USA Today* online, October 2, 2009 (updated August 10, 2010), http://www.usatoday.com/news/health/2009-09-30-drug-overdose_N.htm.

15 Barry Meier, "When Pain Drugs Hurt: Focusing on Doctors," *New York Times*, CNBC online, July 29, 2010, http://www.cnbc.com/id/38464522.

16 "Suspect Charged in Somer Thompson's Murder; Recovering Addict Explains Doctor Shopping," transcript, *Issues with Jane Velez-Mitchell*, March 26, 2010, http://transcripts.cnn.com/TRANSCRIPTS/1003/26/ijvm.01.html.

17 "Lindsay Lohan Starts Serving Jail Sentence," Associated Press, July 20, 2010, http://cbs11tv.com/national/Lindsay.Lohan.jail.2.1814144.html.

18 "Lindsay Lohan Probation Report Released," Radaronline.com, July 7, 2010, http://www.radaronline.com/sites/radaronline.com/files/Lindsay%20Lohan%20Probationc.pdf.

19 Ibid.

20 Letter from Lisa Bloom for the Bloomfirm, Attorneys at Law, to Edmund G. Brown, Jr., Attorney General, California Department of Justice, dated July 28, 2010.

21 United States Department of Health and Human Services Testimony by William K. Hubbard on the Domestic Sale of Prescription Drugs over the Internet, March 27, 2003, http://www.hhs.gov/asl/testify/t030327b.html.

22 Peter Singer, *The Life You Can Save: How to Do Your Part to End World Poverty*, Published by Random House Trade Paperbacks, Reprint Edition, September 14, 2010, page 27.

23 Youtube.com, March 18, 2009. http://www.youtube.com/watch?v=Uv2hS_NulHU.

24 The Henry K. Kaiser Family Foundation Report on Impact of Direct-to-Consumer Advertising on Prescription Drug Spending, June 2003, http://www.kff.org/rxdrugs/6084-index.cfm.

25 "Top 10 Best-Selling Prescription Drugs in America," Listafterlist.com, http://www.listafterlist.com/tabid/57/listid/10716/Health/Top+10+BestSelling+Prescription+Drugs+in+America.aspx.

26 "Bitter Medicine: Pills, Profit and the Public Health," May 29 (no year), http://levine.sscnet.ucla.edu/archive/bitter-medicine.htm.

27 Stephanie Saul, "More Celebrities Finding Roles as Antidepressant Advocates," *New York Times*, March 21, 2005, http://www.nytimes.com/2005/03/21/business/media/21bracco.html.

28 Ibid.

29 John Morgan, "Terry Bradshaw's Winning Drive Against Depression," *USA Today*, January 30, 2004, http://www.usatoday.com/news/health/spotlighthealth/2004-01-30bradshaw_x.htm.

30 Stephanie Saul, "More Celebrities Finding Roles as Antidepressant Advocates," *New York Times*, March 21, 2005, http://www.nytimes.com/2005/03/21/business/media/21bracco.html.

31 Julie Creswell, "Nothing Sells Like Celebrity," *New York Times*, June 22, 2008, http://www.nytimes.com/2008/06/22/business/media/22celeb.html.

32 Melody Petersen, "CNN to Reveal When Guests Promote Drugs for Companies," *New York Times*, August 23, 2002, http://www.nytimes.com/2002/08/23/business/media/23DRUG.html?pagewanted=1&pagewanted=print.

33 Dennis Cauchon, "FDA Advisers Tied to Industry," *USA Today*, September 25, 2000, http://www.commondreams.org/headlines/092500-01.htm. Original links at http://www.usatoday.com/news/washington/2007-03-21-fda-conflicts-interest_N.htm; and http://www.fda.gov/oc/advisory/factsheet080408.html.

34 "Bitter Medicine: Pills, Profit and the Public Health," May 29 (no year), http://levine.sscnet.ucla.edu/archive/bitter-medicine.htm.

35 Duff Wilson, "Poor Children Likelier to Get Antipsychotics," *New York Times*, December 11, 2009, http://www.nytimes.com/2009/12/12/health/12medicaid.html.

36 Jennifer Ashton, M.D., "5 Drugs Kids Steal Most Often from Parents," CBS online, May 7, 2009, http://www.cbsnews.com/stories/2009/05/07/earlyshow/health/main4998006.shtml.

37 Join Together Research Summary, October 30, 2006, http://www.jointogether.org/news/research/summaries/2006/prescription-painkillers.html.

38 Jennifer Ashton, M.D., "5 Drugs Kids Steal Most Often from Parents," CBS online, May 7, 2009, http://www.cbsnews.com/stories/2009/05/07/earlyshow/health/main4998006.shtml.

39 "Teen Trend: 'Cabinet Parties,'" MomLogic.com, March 26, 2010, http://www.momlogic.com/2010/03/teen_trend_cabinet_parties.php.

40 "Brittany Murphy's Mom: My Daughter Didn't Do Drugs," *People*, January 16, 2010, http://www.people.com/people/article/0,,20337389,00.html.

41 Ken Lee, "Brittany Murphy Died from Drug Intoxication and Pneumonia," *People*, February 4, 2010, http://www.people.com/people/article/0,,20341643,00.html.

Chapter 3: The Cybers

1 Dungeons and Dragons website, https://trial.turbine.com/ddo.php?ftui=DDODefault&utm_source=Google_S_DDO&utm_medium=Text&utm_campaign=DDOLaunch0Test&referral=127284&gclid=CMWW2oTbvKICFUJx5Qodam1J5Q.

2 "Parents Neglect Starved Babies to Feed Video Game Addiction," Associated Press, July 14, 2007, http://www.foxnews.com/story/0,2933,289331,00.html.

3 Ryan Van Cleave, foreword to *Unplugged: My Journey into the Dark World of Video Game Addiction* (Deerfield Beach, FL: HCI, 2010), viii.

4 "What is the total number of websites on Internet?" AbhiSays.com, December 29, 2009, http://abhisays.com/internet/what-is-the-total-number-of-websites-on-internet.html.

5 Dan Kadlec, "World Series of Poker: Attack of the Math Brats," *Time*, June 28, 2010, http://www.time.com/time/magazine/article/0,9171,1997467,00.html.

6 Gambling Facts and Statistics, http://overcominggambling.com/gambling-facts.html.

7 Dr. Kimberly Young, "What is Cybersexual Addiction?" HealthyPlace: American's Mental

Health Channel, December 15, 2008, http://www.healthyplace.com/addictions/center-for-internet-addiction-recovery/what-is-cybersexual-addiction/menu-id-1105.

8 Miguel Helft, "For X-Rated, a Domain of Their Own," *New York Times*, June 25, 2010, http://www.nytimes.com/2010/06/26/technology/26domain.html?src=busln.

9 Adult Videochat, Wikipedia, http://en.wikipedia.org/wiki/Adult_video_chat.

10 Online dating service, Wikipedia, http://en.wikipedia.org/wiki/Online_dating_service; and Robert L. Mitchell, "Online dating: It's bigger than porn," Computerworld, February 13, 2009, http://blogs.computerworld.com/online_dating_its_bigger_than_porn.

11 "The Couch-Potato Generation, Kaiser Family Foundation Study," *Time*, February 1, 2010, http://www.time.com/time/magazine/article/0,9171,1955582-2,00.html.

12 "Third of Teens with Phones Text 100 Times a day," Reuters, April 20, 2010, http://www.reuters.com/article/idUSTRE63J0K220100420.

13 Clive Thompson, "Brave New World of Digital Intimacy," *New York Times*, September 5, 2008, http://www.nytimes.com/2008/09/07/magazine/07awareness-t.html?pagewanted=all.

14 Hilary Stout, "Antisocial Networking?" *New York Times*, April 30, 2010, http://www.nytimes.com/2010/05/02/fashion/02BEST.html.

15 Transcript of Text Messages on Wayne Treacy's Phone, *Sun Sentinel*, May 14, 2010, http://www.palmbeachpost.com/news/transcript-of-text-messages-on-wayne-treacys-phone-687916.html and Sue Scheff, "Text Messages Released: Wayne Treacy planned to Snap (Josie Ratley) Neck and then Stomp Her Skull," *Examiner*, May 13, 2010, http://www.examiner.com/parenting-teens-in-fort-lauderdale/text-messages-released-wayne-treacy-planned-to-snap-her-josie-ratley-neck-then-stomp-her-skull.

16 Jan Hoffman, "Online Bullies Pull Schools In," *New York Times*, June 27, 2010, http://www.nytimes.com/2010/06/28/style/28bully.html to the Fray.

17 Ibid.

18 Tamar Lewin, "Teenage Insults Scrawled on Web, Not on Walls," *New York Times*, May 5, 2010, http://www.nytimes.com/2010/05/06/us/06formspring.html.

19 "Alexis Pilkington Brutally Cyber Bullied, Even After Her Suicide," CBS, March 26, 2010, http://www.cbsnews.com/8301-504083_162-20001181-504083.html?tag=content-Main;contentBody; and Oren Yaniv, "Long Island teen's suicide linked to cruel cyber bullies, formspring.me site: police," *New York Daily News*, March 25, 2010, http://www.nydailynews.com/news/ny_crime/2010/03/25/2010-0325_li_teens_suicide_linked_to_cruel_cyberbullies_police.html

20 Alastair Sweeny, *BlackBerry Planet: The Story of Research in Motion and the Little Device that Took the World by Storm* (New York: Wiley, 2009), Kindle location, 2973.

21 Tom Lutz, *Doing Nothing: A History of Loafers, Loungers, Slackers, and Bums in America* (New York: Farrar, Straus and Giroux, 2007), 41.

22 Ram Dass, *Remember, Be Here Now* (Santa Fe, NM: Hanuman Foundation, 1971).

Chapter 4: The Stargazers

1 Sharon Clott, "Was Lady Gaga's VMA Meat Dress Real?" MTV.com, September 13, 2010, http://style.mtv.com/2010/09/13/2010-vmas-was-lady-gagas-meat-dress-real/; and Tim Teeman, "Lady Gaga's meat dress the must-have Halloween costume," *Adelaide Now*, October 22, 2010, http://www.adelaidenow.com.au/entertainment/lady-gagas-meat-dress-the-must-have-halloween-costume/story-e6fredpu-1225942315873.

2 "Starvation for Sanjaya: A Hunger Strike," YouTube.com, http://www.youtube.com/watch?v=YDviPoXJl28&feature=player_embedded.

3 "In Pictures: The Web Celeb 25," Forbes.com, http://www.forbes.com/2010/02/02/web-celebrities-internet-thought-leaders-25_slide_9.html.

4 Tila Tequila "I Love U" music video snippet, YouTube.com, http://www.youtube.com/watch?v=jyt5PA4v0wc.

5 Spike Guys' Choice Awards, Wikipedia, http://en.wikipedia.org/wiki/Spike_Guys'_Choice_Awards.

6 Tila Tequila, Wikipedia, http://en.wikipedia.org/wiki/Tila_Tequila.

7 "3 Year Old Crying Over Justin Bieber," Youtube.com, http://www.youtube.com/watch?v=dTCm8tdHkfI.

8 *Issues with Jane Velez-Mitchell* transcript, Headline News Channel, July 6, 2010, http://transcripts.cnn.com/TRANSCRIPTS/1007/06/ijvm.01.html.

9 Alexandra Petri, "Why is America Googling Lindsay Lohan's fingernail?," *Washington Post*, July 7, 2010, http://voices.washingtonpost.com/postpartisan/2010/07/why_is_america_googling_lindsa.html.

10 Bryan Walsh, "The Electrifying Edison," *Time*, June 23, 2010, http://www.time.com/time/specials/packages/article/0,28804,1999143_1999200,00.html.

11 Deborah Sontag, "In Haiti, the Displaced Are Left Clinging to the Edge," *New York Times*, July 10, 2010, http://www.nytimes.com/2010/07/11/world/americas/11haiti.html.

12 "Gibson's Anti-Semitic Tirade—Alleged Cover Up," TMZ Staff, July 28, 2006, http://www.tmz.com/2006/07/28/gibsons-anti-semitic-tirade-alleged-cover-up.

13 Michael Cieply, "Stars, Cameras and Theatrics Strain Courts," *New York Times*, July 9, 2010, http://www.nytimes.com/2010/07/10/us/10celebrity.html.

14 Sam Vaknin, Ph.D., *Malignant Self Love*, http://samvak.tripod.com/faq19.html.

15 Drew Pinsky, M.D., *The Mirror Effect: How Celebrity Narcissism Is Seducing America* (New York: Harper, 2009), 6.

16 "Julia Roberts stuns yogurt shop customers," *New York Post*, March 23, 2010, http://www.nypost.com/p/pagesix/earthly_visit_Jnj1il6hH7HFkYRxxnkcFO.

17 YourDictionary.com, http://www.yourdictionary.com/venerate.

18 Luchina Fisher, "Obsessive Fan of Paula Abdul Commits Suicide," ABC News, November 13, 2008, http://abcnews.go.com/Entertainment/story?id=6241069&page=1.

19 Ibid.

Chapter 5: The Players

1 Inbar, Michael, "Admitted Tiger Mistress: No $, Only Heartbreak," *Today Show*, December 11, 2009, http://today.msnbc.msn.com/id/34376988.

2 Cristine Everette, "Tiger Woods Was Nicknamed 'Urkel' by Teammates on His College Golf Team," *New York Daily News*, April 13, 2010, http://www.nydailynews.com/gossip/2010/04/13/2010-0413_tiger_woods_was_nicknamed_urkel_by_teammates_on_his_college_golf_team.html.

3 *Sex and Love Addicts Anonymous: The Basic Text for The Augustine Fellowship*, published by the Augustine Fellowship, June 1986, p. 47.

4 Keith Morrison, "Dateline NBC: Battling sexual addiction," NBC News, February 24, 2004, http://www.msnbc.msn.com/id/4302347.

5 Bill Maher, "New Rule: Stop Saying 'Sex Addict' Like It's a Bad Thing," *Huffington Post*, February 26, 2010, http://www.huffingtonpost.com/bill-maher/new-rule-stop-saying-sex_b_478545.html.

6 Keith Morrison, "Dateline NBC: Battling sexual addiction," NBC News, February 24, 2004, http://www.msnbc.msn.com/id/4302347.

7 *Sex and Love Addicts Anonymous: The Basic Text for The Augustine Fellowship*, published by the Augustine Fellowship, June 1986, p. 34.

8 Keith Morrison, "Dateline NBC: Battling sexual addiction," NBC News, February 24, 2004, http://www.msnbc.msn.com/id/4302347.

9 Lisa DePaulo, "Hello America, My Name Is Rielle Hunter," *GQ*, April 2010, http://www.gq.com/news-politics/politics/201004/rielle-hunter-john-edwards-exclusive-interview.

10 Brenda Shaeffer, *Is It Love or Is It Addiction?* 2nd ed. (Center City, MN: Hazelden, 1997), 25 and 26.

11 Lisa DePaulo, "Hello America, My Name Is Rielle Hunter," *GQ*, April 2010, http://www.gq.com/news-politics/politics/201004/rielle-hunter-john-edwards-exclusive-interview.

12 Mark Langford, "Family Life 'Best Thing Ever' for Tiger Woods," Sky News Online, December 15, 2009, http://news.sky.com/skynews/Home/World-News/Golf-Star-Tiger-Woods-Praised-Family-In-Last-TV-Interview-Before-Scandal-As-Cori-Rist-Claims-Affair/Article/200912315500700.

13 "Tiger Apologizes, Heads Back to Therapy," transcript, *Issues with Jane Velez-Mitchell*, February 19, 2010, http://transcripts.cnn.com/TRANSCRIPTS/1002/19/ijvm.01.html.

14 Rebecca Leung, "Porn in the U.S.A.: Steve Kroft Reports on a $10 Billion Industry," September 5, 2004, http://www.cbsnews.com/stories/2003/11/21/60minutes/main585049.shtml.

15 Theatrical Market Statistics. Motion Picture Association of America, 2009, http://mpaa.org/Resources/091af5d6-faf7-4f58-9a8e-405466c1c5e5.pdf and "Statistics on Pornography, Sexual Addiction and Online Perpetrators," SafeFamilies.org, http://www.safefamilies.org/sfStats.php.

16 "Statistics on Pornography, Sexual Addiction and Online Perpetrators," SafeFamilies.org, http://www.safefamilies.org/sfStats.php.

17 Rebecca Leung, "Porn in the U.S.A.: Steve Kroft Reports on a $10 Billion Industry," September 5, 2004, http://www.cbsnews.com/stories/2003/11/21/60minutes/main585049.shtml.

18 Ibid.; and Frank Rich, "Naked Capitalists: There's No Business Like Porn Business," *New York Times*, May 20, 2001, http://www.nytimes.com/2001/05/20/magazine/20PORN.html.

19 Rebecca Leung, "Porn in the U.S.A.: Steve Kroft Reports on a $10 Billion Industry," September 5, 2004, http://www.cbsnews.com/stories/2003/11/21/60minutes/main585049.shtml.

20 "Somer Thompson Murder: Person of Interest Jarred Harrell Arrested with Child Porno," CBS News, February 12, 2010, http://www.cbsnews.com/8301-504083_162-6139219-504083.html.

21 Arrest Warrant, Jarred Mitchell Harrell, February 10, 2010.

22 Affidavit for Arrest Warrant, Jarred Mitchell Harrell, February 25, 2010, http://download.gannett.edgesuite.net/wtsp/pdfs/2010/0301210_Harrell1.PDF.

23 "Suspect Charged in Somer Thompson's Murder," transcript, *Issues with Jane Velez-Mitchell*, March 26, 2010, http://archives.cnn.com/TRANSCRIPTS/1003/26/ijvm.01.html; and Arrest Warrant in the Name of the State of Florida, February 10, 2010, http://www.actionnewsjax.com/media/lib/1/a/9/d/a9da06ab-10f5-47f1-956d-30375e288939/CP_Warrant.pdf.

24 "Suspect Charged in Somer Thompson's Murder," transcript, *Issues with Jane Velez-Mitchell*, March 26, 2010, http://archives.cnn.com/TRANSCRIPTS/1003/26/ijvm.01.html.

25 Michele McPhee, Lauren Pearle, and Yunji De Nies, "16 Pairs of Women's Underwear Found in Home of Alleged 'Craigslist Killer,'" ABC News, April 29, 2009, http://abcnews.go.com/print?id=7464224.

26 "The Craigslist Killer: Seven Days of Rage; '48 Hours' Examines the Latest Developments in the Case Against Accused 'Craigslist Killer, Philip Markoff'" *48 Hours/Mystery*, July 10, 2010, http://www.cbsnews.com/stories/2010/07/10/48hours/main6666324_page4.shtml?tag=contentMain;contentBody.

Chapter 6: The Bloodlusters

1 Elliot Spagat, "John Gardner Charged in Chelsea King Case," *Huffington Post*, March 3, 2010, http://www.huffingtonpost.com/2010/03/03/john-gardner-sex-offender_n_484374.html.

2 Statement of the case, People Sentencing Memorandum, Superior Court of the State of California, San Diego, August 24, 2010, http://www.scribd.com/doc/28122193/2000-Sentencing-Memorandum-for-John-Gardner.

3 "Body Found Believed to be Missing Teen Jogger," transcript, *Issues with Jane Velez-Mitchell*, March 2, 2010, http://archives.cnn.com/TRANSCRIPTS/1003/02/ijvm.01.html.

4 Tony Perry, "John Gardner sentenced to life for killing Amber Dubois and Chelsea King," *Los Angeles Times*, May 14, 2010, http://latimesblogs.latimes.com/lanow/2010/05/john-gardner-sentenced-chelsea-king-amber-dubois.html.

5 "Estimates of A.A. Groups and Members," Alcoholics Anonymous website, 2010, http://www.aa.org/subpage.cfm?page=74.

6 Cathy Cockrell, "Arrest of kidnap suspect Phillip Garrido hinged on instincts and diligence of two members of UC Berkeley police force," UC Berkeley News Center, August 28, 2009, http://berkeley.edu/news/media/releases/2009/08/28_ucpd.shtml.

7 Sam Stanton, "Parole agents rarely checked on Garrido in early years, documents show," *Sacramento Bee*, April 16, 2010, http://www.sacbee.com/2010/04/16/2684665/parole-agents-rarely-checked-on.html.

8 Robert J. Lopez, "Parole agents talked to but did not identify Dugard, report says," *Los Angeles Times*, July 8, 2010, http://articles.latimes.com/2010/jul/08/local/la-me-0708-parole-dugard-20100708.

9 Rampton Secure Hospital is a high-security psychiatric hospital near the village of Woodbeck between Retford and Rampton in the Bassetlaw District of Nottinghamshire, England.

10 Tony Perry, "John Gardner sentenced to life for killing Amber Dubois and Chelsea King," *Los Angeles Times*, May 14, 2010, http://latimesblogs.latimes.com/lanow/2010/05/john-gardner-sentenced-chelsea-king-amber-dubois.html.

11 Eugene V. Beresin, M.D., "The Impact of Media Violence on Children and Adolescents," American Academy of Child and Adolescent Psychiatry, http://www.aacap.org/cs/root/developmentor/the_impact_of_media_violence_on_children_and_adolescents_opportunities_for_clinical_interventions; and Senate Committee on the Judiciary, "Children, violence, and the media: A report for parents and policy makers," September 14, 1999. Reprinted at http://www.kidsfirst.org/articles-info/violence.htm.

12 George Gerbner, author of "Reclaiming our Cultural Mythology," http://www.context.org/ICLIB/IC38/Gerbner.htm.

13 Expanded Homicide Data, Table 1, Murder by race and sex 2009, U.S. Department of Justice/FBI, http://www.fbi.gov/about-us/cjis/ucr/crime-in-the-u.s/2009.

14 "FBI: Murder, Violent Crime Dropped in 2008; Number of Reported Rapes Lowest in 20 Years; Property Crimes Decline Overall, But Burglaries, Larceny-Thefts Go Up," CBS/AP, Sept. 15, 2009, http://www.cbsnews.com/stories/2009/09/14/national/main5309836.shtml.

Chapter 7: The Punishers

1 DeJarion Echols Profile, Families Against Mandatory Minimums, http://www.famm.org/ProfilesofInjustice/FederalProfiles/DeJarionEchols.aspx.

2 "I Wasn't Driving, the Black Kid Was," TMZ.com, July 27, 2007, http://www.tmz.com/2007/07/27/lindsay-i-wasnt-driving-the-black-kid-was.

3 Tracy Connor, "Inside LiLo's Crazy Ride from Hell," *New York Daily News*, July 28, 2007, http://

www.nydailynews.com/gossip/2007/07/28/2007-07-28_inside_lilos_crazy_ride_from_hell.html.

4 Mike Fleeman, "Lindsay Lohan Sued Over Car Chase," People.com, August 14, 2007, http://www.people.com/people/article/0,,20051654,00.html.

5 "Lohan Charged With 7 Misdemeanor DUI Counts," CBS, August 23, 2007, http://cbs2.com/local/Lindsay.Lohan.DUI.2.534912.html. Accessed 8/18/10.

6 Rich Shapiro, "Michael Douglas' son, Cameron Douglas, pleads guilty to drug trafficking charges," New York Daily News, January 27, 2010, http://www.nydailynews.com/gossip/2010/01/27/2010-01-27_michael_douglas_son_cameron_douglas_pleads_guilty_to_drug_trafficking_charges.html.

7 Ibid and Charlotte Triggs, "Michael Douglas: Prison Will Help My Son 'Start Afresh,'" People.com, May 3, 2010, http://www.people.com/people/article/0,,20365938,00.html.

8 "Cameron Douglas Turned In Drug Suppliers to Get Lesser Sentence, Report Says," Fox News.com, July 26, 2010, http://www.foxnews.com/entertainment/2010/07/26/cameron-douglas-turned-drug-suppliers-lesser-sentence.

9 CNN Wire Staff, "Obama signs bill reducing cocaine sentencing gap," CNN, August 3, 2010, http://www.cnn.com/2010/POLITICS/08/03/fair.sentencing/index.html.

10 "Frequently Asked Questions: The Fair Sentencing Act of 2010," Families Against Mandatory Minimums, http://www.famm.org.

11 U.S. Census Quickfacts, 2009, http://quickfacts.census.gov/qfd/states/00000.html; and Pierre Thomas and Jason Ryan, "U.S. Prison Population Hits All-Time High: 2.3 Million Incarcerated," ABC News, June 6, 2008, http://abcnews.go.com/TheLaw/story?id=5009270&page=1.

12 "List of Countries by Population," Wikipedia, http://en.wikipedia.org/wiki/List_of_countries_by_population.

13 "World Prison Population List," 8th ed., http://www.kcl.ac.uk/depsta/law/research/icps/downloads/wppl-8th_41.pdf; and Adam Liptak, "1 in 100 U.S. Adults Behind Bars, New Study Says," New York Times, February 28, 2008, http://www.nytimes.com/2008/02/28/us/28cnd-prison.html.

14 Probation and Parole in the United States, 2006, U.S. Department of Justice, http://bjs.ojp.usdoj.gov/content/pub/pdf/ppus06.pdf.

15 Dominick Dunne, The Way We Lived Then: Recollections of a Well-Known Name Dropper (New York: Crown, 1999), 192–193. and "Sharon Tate," Wikipedia, http://en.wikipedia.org/wiki/Sharon_Tate#cite_note-dominickdunne-17.

16 Joan Didion, The White Album (Farrar, Straus and Giroux: 1990), 47.

17 Travis Pratt, Addicted to Incarceration: Corrections Policy and the Politics of Misinformation in the United States (Thousand Oaks, CA: Sage Publications: 2008), 6, 75.

18 "David Berkowitz," Wikipedia, http://en.wikipedia.org/wiki/David_Berkowitz#Psychological_profile_and_other_police_investigations and Corky Siemaszko, "The Summer," New York Daily News, http://www.nydailynews.com/features/sonofsam/summer.html.

19 Elizabeth Alexander, "Michigan Breaks the Political Logjam: A New Model for Reducing Prison Populations," American Civil Liberties Union, November 2009, 3, http://www.aclu.org/files/assets/2009-12-18-MichiganReport.pdf.

20 Michael Myser, "The Hard Sell," CNNMoney.com, March 15, 2007, http://money.cnn.com/magazines/business2/business2_archive/2006/12/01/8394995/index.htm.

21 Ibid.

22 James J. Stephan, "State Prison Expenditures 2001," Bureau of Justice Statistics, http://bjs.ojp.usdoj.gov/content/pub/pdf/spe01.pdf.

23 Michael Myser, "The Hard Sell," CNNMoney.com, March 15, 2007, http://money.cnn.com/magazines/business2/business2_archive/2006/12/01/8394995/index.htm.

24 Corrections Corporation of America, http://www.correctionscorp.com/about.

25 Ibid.

26 "U.S. Prison Labor Output: $2.4 Billion Annually," Democratic Leadership Council, August 26, 2009, http://www.dlc.org/ndol_ci.cfm?kaid=108&subid=900003&contentid=255055.

27 UNICOR Federal Prison Industries, Inc., Federal Bureau of Prisons, http://www.bop.gov/inmate_programs/unicor.jsp.

28 Ibid.

29 Vicky Pelaez, "The Prison Industry in the United States: Big Business or a New Form of Slavery?" GlobalResearch.ca., March 10, 2008, http://www.globalresearch.ca/index.php?context=va&aid=8289.

30 "Prisoners Allowed to Work Jobs with Access to Social Security Numbers," *Jacksonville Observer*, March 18, 2010, http://www.jaxobserver.com/2010/03/18/prisoners-allowed-to-work-jobs-with-access-to-social-security-numbers.

31 UNICOR Annual Report, 2008, page 12, http://www.unicor.gov/information/publications/pdfs/corporate/catar2008_C.pdf

32 Vicky Pelaez, "The Prison Industry in the United States: Big Business or a New Form of Slavery?" GlobalResearch.ca., March 10, 2008, http://www.globalresearch.ca/index.php?context=va&aid=8289.

33 Kevin Johnson, "Commission Warns of Harm Isolation Can Do to Prisoners," *USA Today*, June 7, 2006, http://www.usatoday.com/news/nation/2006-06-07-solitary-confinement-study_x.htm.

34 Pete du Pont, "Should Prisoners be Allowed to Work?" National Center for Policy Analysis, November 29, 1995, http://www.ncpa.org/commentaries/should-prisoners-be-allowed-to-work.

35 Caroline Winter, "What Do Prisoners Make for Victoria's Secret?" *Mother Jones*, July/August 2008, http://motherjones.com/politics/2008/07/what-do-prisoners-make-victorias-secret.

36 Victor Perlo, "Prison Labor in the U.S.," marxism-news@lists.econ.utah.edu, August 17, 1999, http://www.hartford-hwp.com/archives/45b/157.html.

37 "Confronting Confinement," Commission on Safety and Abuse in America's Prisons, June 8, 2006, http://www.prisoncommission.org.

38 Travis Pratt, *Addicted to Incarceration: Corrections Policy and the Politics of Misinformation in the United States* (Thousand Oaks, CA: Sage Publications, 2008), 93.

39 Christopher J. Mumola, "Incarcerated Parents and Their Children," U.S. Department of Justice Bureau of Justice Statistics (Washington, DC: U.S. Department of Justice, August 2000), 2. Cited by Get the Facts/DrugWarFacts.org, http://www.drugwarfacts.org/cms/node/64; and "Children of Incarcerated Children," Council on Crime and Justice, January 2006, http://www.racialdisparity.org/files/CCJ%20CIP%20FINAL%20REPORT.pdf and "Parents in Prison and their Minor Children," Bureau of Justice Statistics, Laura E. Glaze and Laura M. Maruschak, August 2008, http://bjs.ojp.usdoj.gov/content/pub/pdf/pptmc.pdf.

40 Patrice Gaines, "The Cost of Incarceration," *Tri-State Defender*, NNPA News Service, October 8, 2009, http://tri-statedefenderonline.com/articlelive/articles/4223/1/The-Curse-of-Mandatory-Minimums/Page1.html.

41 David Von Drehle, "What's Behind America's Falling Crime Rate," *Time*, February 22, 2010, http://www.time.com/time/magazine/article/0,9171,1963761,00.html.

42 Jeremy Hubbard, "Outrage Follows Arrest in Rape of 7-Year-Old New Jersey Girl," ABC World News, April 4, 2010, http://Abcnews.go.com/WN/charged-trenton-gang-rape-year/story?id=10283128.

Chapter 8: The Breeders

1 "First Two Octuplets Come Home from Hospital, Intensifying Mother Nadya Suleman's Star Status," Associated Press, March 18, 2009, http://www.foxnews.com/story/0,2933,509616,00.html.

2 Ibid.

3 *Issues with Jane Velez-Mitchell*, transcript, CNN.com, March 18, 2009, http://transcripts.cnn.com/TRANSCRIPTS/0903/18/ijvm.01.html.

4 "Octo-Mom: 'I Just Kept Going,'" Associated Press/NBC Los Angeles, February 7, 2009, http://www.nbclosangeles.com/news/local-beat/Octuplets-Mom-Released-from-Hospital-Babies-Stay.html; and Dan Childs, Alice Gomstyn, Jim Vojtech, and Chris Fancescani, "Octuplets' Mom: Can She Afford to Raise 14 Kids?" ABC News, February 2, 2009, http://abcnews.go.com/Health/WomensHealth/story?id=6774471&page=1.

5 Kimi Yoshino and Jessica Garrison, "Octuplets could be costly for taxpayers," *Los Angeles Times*, February 11, 2009, http://articles.latimes.com/2009/feb/11/local/me-octuplets11.

6 Ibid.

7 "Octo-Mom: 'I Just Kept Going,'" Associated Press/NBC Los Angeles, February 7, 2009, http://www.nbclosangeles.com/news/local-beat/Octuplets-Mom-Released-from-Hospital-Babies-Stay.html.

8 *Issues with Jane Velez-Mitchell*, transcript, CNN.com, March 18, 2009, http://transcripts.cnn.com/TRANSCRIPTS/0903/18/ijvm.01.html.

9 Ibid.

10 "A Century of Change: America, 1900–1999," U.S. Census Bureau, https://www.msu.edu/~bsilver/pls440century.html.

11 Lester R. Brown, Brian Halweil, and Gary Gardner, *Beyond Malthus: Nineteen Dimensions of the Population Challenge* (New York: W.W. Norton, 1999), 17.

12 Ibid.

13 "Octo-Mom: 'I Just Kept Going,'" Associated Press/NBC Los Angeles, February 7, 2009, http://www.nbclosangeles.com/news/local-beat/Octuplets-Mom-Released-from-Hospital-Babies-Stay.html.

14 Barry Wigmore, "I wanted a huge family to make up for my lonely childhood: Mother of octuplets speaks for the first time," *Daily Mail*, February 7, 2009, http://www.dailymail.co.uk/news/worldnews/article-1137273/I-wanted-huge-family-make-lonely-childhood-Mother-octuplets-speaks-time.html.

15 Martha Brockenbrough, "Can You Be Addicted to Pregnancy? When Pregnancy Becomes the Focus of Your Life," *Women'sHealth*, July/August 2009, http://www.womenshealthmag.com/health/pregnancy-perks.

16 United States Population Projections: 2000–2050, U.S. Census Bureau, http://www.census.gov/population/www/projections/usinterimproj/idbsummeth.html.

17 Dave Tilford, "Why Consumption Matters," Sierra Club, http://www.sierraclub.org/sustainable_consumption/tilford.asp; and United Nations Development Programme, Human Development Report, 1998, http://hdr.undp.org/en/reports/global/hdr1998.

18 U.S. Census Bureau, 2006–2008 American Community Survey 3-Year Estimates, http://factfinder.census.gov/servlet/ACSSAFFFacts.

19 The World Factbook, Central Intelligence Agency, https://www.cia.gov/library/publications/the-world-factbook/rankorder/2127rank.html; and Total Fertility UNdata, http://data.un.org/Data.aspx?d=PopDiv&f=variableID%3A54.

20 "More Babies Born in 2007 Than Any Other Year in U.S. History," Associated Press, March 19, 2009, http://www.foxnews.com/story/0,2933,509672,00.html; and Sharon

Jayson, "Is this the next baby boom?" *USA Today*, July 17, 2008, http://www.usatoday.com/news/nation/2008-07-16-baby-boomlet_N.htm.

21 Martha Brockenbrough, "Can You Be Addicted to Pregnancy? When Pregnancy Becomes the Focus of Your Life," *Women'sHealth*, July/August 2009, http://www.womenshealth-mag.com/health/pregnancy-perks; and "More Babies Born in 2007 Than Any Other Year in U.S. History," Associated Press, March 19, 2009, http://www.foxnews.com/story/0,2933,509672,00.html.

22 "Mortality Trends in the USA, Main Category: HIV/AIDS," *Medical News Today*, February 28, 2004, http://www.medicalnewstoday.com/articles/6219.php.

23 Haya El Nasser, "U.S. Hispanic population to triple by 2050," *USA Today*, February, 12, 2008, http://www.usatoday.com/news/nation/2008-02-11-population-study_N.htm and "Humanae Vitae," Encyclical Letter by Pope John Paul VI, July 25, 1968, http://www.vatican.va/holy_father/paul_vi/encyclicals/documents/hf_p-vi_enc_25071968_humanae-vitae_en.html.

24 "FACTSHEET: Hunger, the world's silent killer," Reuters, September 15, 2005, http://www.alertnet.org/thefacts/reliefresources/112679705053.htm.

25 Neale Donald Walsch, *Conversations with God: An Uncommon Dialogue (Book 1)*, 1st ed. (New York: Putnam Adult, 1996), 49.

26 World Orphans Day, http://www.worldorphansday.com.

27 Jason Kovacs, "Orphan Statistics" ABBA Fund, October 16, 2009, http://abbafund.wordpress.com/2009/07/27/how-many-orphans-are-there-update/; and Help End Local Poverty, http://www.helpendlocalpoverty.com/2009/10/orphan-statistics.

28 Adam Nossiter, "Famine Persist in Niger, but Denial is Past," *New York Times*, May 3, 2010, http://www.nytimes.com/2010/05/04/world/africa/04niger.html.

29 The World Factbook, Central Intelligence Agency, https://www.cia.gov/library/publications/the-world-factbook/rankorder/2127rank.html.

30 "AIDS epidemic update, 2009." UNAIDS, Joint United Nations Programme on HIV/AIDS, http://data.unaids.org:80/pub/Report/2009/JC1700_Epi_Update_2009_en.pdf.

31 Donald G. McNeil Jr., "At Front Lines, AIDS War Is Falling Apart," *New York Times*, May 9, 2010, http://www.nytimes.com/2010/05/10/world/africa/10aids.html?pagewanted=print.

32 Joel E. Cohen, *How Many People Can the Earth Support?* (New York: W.W. Norton, 1996), 374.

33 Lester R. Brown, Brian Halweil, and Gary Gardner, *Beyond Malthus: Nineteen Dimensions of the Population Challenge* (New York: W.W. Norton, 1999), 131.

34 Marc Santora, "Negligent Upstate Couple Is Told Not to Procreate," *New York Times*, May 11, 2004, http://www.nytimes.com/2004/05/11/nyregion/11couple.html.

35 Ann Hoevel, "Overpopulation could be people, planet problem," CNN, April 8, 2008, http://www.cnn.com/2007/TECH/science/09/25/overpopulation.overview/index.html.

36 John Robbins, "2,500 Gallons All Wet?" EarthSave, http://www.earthsave.org/environment/water.htm; Jeff Nelson, "8,500 Gallons of Water for 1 Pound of Beef," Vegsource, http://www.vegsource.com/articles2/water_stockholm.htm; and "Beef: Environment—Water Concerns," *New American Dream*, http://www.newdream.org/food/beef_water1.php.

Chapter 9: The Gluttons

1 Elizabeth Medes, "In The U.S., Obesity Levels Remain High but Stable in 2010," Gallup. October 8, 2010, http://www.gallup.com/poll/143483/Obesity-Levels-Remain-High-Stable 2010.aspx?utm_source=tagrss&utm_medium=rss&utm_campaign=syndication&utm_term=Well-Being%20Index.

2 Bonnie Erbe, "Are Fat TV Shows Empowering or Exploitative?" CBS News, July 28, 2009, http://www.cbsnews.com/stories/2009/07/29/usnews/whispers/main5196252.shtml.

3 David K. LI, "Director 'fed' Up," *New York Post*, February 17, 2010, http://www.nypost.com/p/news/national/director_fed_up_syAY2YA2MaFsIhxq3Ve0RJ.

4 Steven Reinberg, "Almost 10 Percent of U.S. Medical Costs Tied to Obesity," HealthDay Reporter, ABC News, July 28, 2010, http://abcnews.go.com/Health/Healthday/story?id=8184975&page=1.

5 Weight-Control Information Network (WIN) statistics, http://www.win.niddk.nih.gov/; and BusinessKnowledgeSource.com, http://www.businessknowledgesource.com/health/how_to_reduce_obesity_in_the_workplace_027924.html.

6 "CDC Downscales Mortality Risk from Obesity, USA," Medical News Today, April 21, 2005, http://www.medicalnewstoday.com/articles/23210.php; and Kaiser Daily Health Policy Report, February 10, 2005, http://www.kaisernetwork.org/daily_reports/rep_index.cfm?hint=3&DR_ID=28091.

7 Rob Stein, "Obesity Passing Smoking as Top Avoidable Cause of Death," *Washington Post*, March 10, 2004, http://www.washingtonpost.com/ac2/wp-dyn/A43253-2004Mar9?language=printer.

8 Bryan Walsh, "Getting Real About the High Price of Cheap Food," *Time*, August 21, 2009, http://www.time.com/time/health/article/0,8599,1917458,00.html.

9 Ibid.

10 Howard Lyman and Glen Merzer, *MAD COWBOY: Plain Truth from the Cattle Rancher Who Won't Eat Meat* (New York: Scribner, 2001).

11 "Americans Are Obsessed with Fast Food: The Dark Side of the All-American Meal," interview with Eric Schlosser, CBS Healthwatch, January 18, 2001, http://www.cbsnews.com/stories/2002/01/31/health/main326858.shtml.

12 "Q&A with Morgan Spurlock," SnagFilms, 2009, http://www.snagfilms.com/films/profile/morgan_spurlock.

13 "Fast Food Nation," Wikipedia, 2010, http://en.wikipedia.org/wiki/Fast_Food_Nation_(film).

14 "Americans Are Obsessed with Fast Food: The Dark Side of the All-American Meal," interview with Eric Schlosser, CBS Healthwatch, January 18, 2001, http://www.cbsnews.com/stories/2002/01/31/health/main326858.shtml.

15 Corky Siemaszko, "Fatty foods may be just as addictive as heroin and cocaine: study," *New York Daily News*, May 29, 2010, http://www.nydailynews.com/lifestyle/2010/03/29/2010-03-29_fatty_foods_may_be_just_as_addictive_as_heroin_and_cocaine_study.html.

16 "Compulsive Eating Shares Addictive Biochemical Mechanism with Cocaine, Heroin Abuse, Study Shows," *ScienceDaily*, March 29, 2010, http://www.sciencedaily.com/releases/2010/03/100328170243.htm.

17 "McDonald's tests a bigger burger, report says," CNNMoney.com, March 7, 2007, http://money.cnn.com/2007/03/07/news/companies/mcdonalds_burger/index.htm; and "Angus Management: McDonald's Intros New Burger Line," BurgerBusiness.com, http://www.burgerbusiness.com/?p=1633.

18 "Americans Are Obsessed with Fast Food: The Dark Side of the All-American Meal," interview with Eric Schlosser, CBS Healthwatch, January 18, 2001, http://www.cbsnews.com/stories/2002/01/31/health/main326858.shtml.

19 T. Colin Campbell and Thomas M. Campbell II, *The China Study* (Dallas: BenBella Books, 2006), http://www.thechinastudy.com/about.html.

20 Jonathan Safran Foer, "The Food Issue: Against Meat," *New York Times*, October 7, 2009, http://www.nytimes.com/2009/10/11/magazine/11foer-t.html?_r=1&pagewanted=all.

21 Diane Brady and Christopher Palmeri, "The Pet Economy," *Bloomberg Businessweek*, August 6, 2007, http://www.businessweek.com/magazine/content/07_32/b4045001.htm.

22 Rebecca Ruiz, "Are You Eating Too Much Meat?" *Forbes* and Associated Press, March 24, 2009, http://www.forbes.com/2009/03/24/eating-red-meat-lifestyle-health-red-meat-study.html.

23 Russell Goldman, "KFC to Honor Oprah's Free Chicken Coupons," ABCNews.com, May 7, 2009, http://abcnews.go.com/Business/story?id=7527626&page=1; and Lisa Respers France, "Oprah coupon craze leaves KFC customers hungry for more," CNN.com, May 8, 2009, http://www.cnn.com/2009/LIVING/05/08/oprah.kfc.coupon/index.html.

24 Neal Barnard, M.D., *Breaking the Food Seduction* (New York: St. Martin's Griffin, 2004), 63. He also cites M. R. Yeomans, P. Wright, H. A. Macleod, and J. A. Critchley, "Effects of nalmefene on feeding in humans," *Psychopharmacology* (1990): 426–32.

25 Mark Bittman, "Rethinking the Meat-Guzzler," *New York Times*, January 27, 2008,http://www.nytimes.com/2008/01/27/weekinreview/27bittman.html.

26 "Rearing cattle produces more greenhouse gases than driving cars, UN report warns," UN News Centre, November 29, 2006, www.un.org/apps/news/story.asp?newsID=20772&CR1=warning.

27 Mark Bittman, "Rethinking the Meat-Guzzler," *New York Times*, January 27, 2008, http://www.nytimes.com/2008/01/27/weekinreview/27bittman.html.

28 Jennifer Viegas, "Gulf Wildlife 'Dead Zone' Keeps Growing," Discovery.com, May 7, 2010, http://news.discovery.com/animals/gulf-dead-zone-oil-spill.html?print=true.

29 Resenberger, B., "Curb on US Waste Urged to Help the Worlds Hungry," *New York Times*, 14 Nov. 1974, http://www.veganworldnetwork.org/topic_environment_meat_eating.php; and in the book: John Robbins, *May All Be Fed: A Diet For A New World:* Including recipes by Jia Patton and Friends (Harper Perennial, October 1, 1993), 38.

30 "W. Virginia town shrugs at being fattest city," Associated Press and MSNBC, November 17, 2008, http://www.msnbc.msn.com/id/27697364.

31 Jordan Lite, "Overweight friends will lard it over," *New York Daily News*, July 26, 2007, http://www.nydailynews.com/lifestyle/health/2007/07/26/2007-07-26_overweight_friends_will_lard_it_over_you.html.

32 Barbara Kantrowitz, "Are Fat Friends Bad for Each Other?" *Newsweek* Web Exclusive, August 24, 2009, http://www.newsweek.com/id/213163.

33 Judi Hollis, *Fat Is a Family Affair*, 2nd ed. (Center City, MN: Hazelden, 2003), introduction.

Chapter 10: The Scrubbers

1 Jessica Haddad, Eric M. Strauss, and David Muir, "Germs: 'No Deal' for Host Howie Mandel," ABC News, November 24, 2009, http://abcnews.go.com/2020/howie-mandel-public-obsessive-compulisve-disorder-fear-germs/story?id=9153966.

2 Ibid.

3 Suellen Hoy, *Chasing Dirt: The American Pursuit of Cleanliness* (New York: Oxford University Press, 1996), 40.

4 "Immigration to the United States," Wikipedia, http://en.wikipedia.org/wiki/Immigration_to_the_United_States; and Jeanette Altarriba and Roberto R. Heredia, *An Introduction to Bilingualism: Principles and Processes* (Philadelphia, PA: Psychology Press, 2008), 212. http://books.google.com/books?id=87snuOaE7DwC&pg=PA212&dq&hl=en#v=onepage&q&f=false.

5 Suellen Hoy, *Chasing Dirt: The American Pursuit of Cleanliness* (New York: Oxford University Press, 1996), 88 and 89.

6 Ibid., 145.

7 Katherine Ashenburg, *The Dirt on Clean: An Unsanitized History* (New York: North Point Press, 2008), 4 and 5.

8 "Imagine a Touchable World," Purell website, http://www.purell.com/page.jhtml?id=/purell/include/reasons.inc.

9 Lyndsey Layton, "FDA Says Studies on Triclosan, Used in Sanitizers and Soaps, Raise Concerns," *Washington Post*, April 8, 2010, http://www.washingtonpost.com/wp-dyn/content/article/2010/04/07/AR2010040704621.html.

10 Lisa Wade McCormick, "Report Warns Against Overuse of Household Disinfectants," ConsumerAffairs.com, November 11, 2009, http://www.consumeraffairs.com/news04/2009/11/disinfectants.html.

11 Lyndsey Layton, "FDA Says Studies on Triclosan, Used in Sanitizers and Soaps, Raise Concerns," Washington Post, April 8, 2010, http://www.washingtonpost.com/wp-dyn/content/article/2010/04/07/AR2010040704621.html.

12 Lisa Wade McCormick, "Report Warns Against Overuse of Household Disinfectants," ConsumerAffairs.com, November 11, 2009, http://www.consumeraffairs.com/news04/2009/11/disinfectants.html; and Alexandra Scranton, *Disinfectant Overkill: How Too Clean May Be Hazardous to Our Health*, Women's Voices for the Earth, November 2009, http://www.womensvoices.org/our-work/safe-cleaning-products/learn-more/disinfectant-overkill/.

13 Lyndsey Layton, "FDA Says Studies on Triclosan, Used in Sanitizers and Soaps, Raise Concerns," *Washington Post*, April 8, 2010, http://www.washingtonpost.com/wp-dyn/content/article/2010/04/07/AR2010040704621.html.

14 "Endocrine System," Wikipedia, http://en.wikipedia.org/wiki/Endocrine_system.

15 Lyndsey Layton, "FDA Says Studies on Triclosan, Used in Sanitizers and Soaps, Raise Concerns," *Washington Post*, April 8, 2010, http://www.washingtonpost.com/wp-dyn/content/article/2010/04/07/AR2010040704621.html.

16 "Antibacterial Cleaners Can Hurt Immune System," ABC News, July 17 (no year), http://abcnews.go.com/Health/story?id=118140&page=1; and Stuart B. Levy, "Antibacterial Household Products: Cause for Concern," presentation from the 2000 Emerging Infectious Diseases Conference in Atlanta, Georgia. Posted on the Centers for Disease Control and Prevention website, http://www.cdc.gov/ncidod/eid/vol7no3_supp/levy.htm.

17 Mark Schapiro, *Exposed: The Toxic Chemistry of Everyday Products and What's at Stake for American Power* (White River Junction, VT: Chelsea Green, 2009), 25.

18 Ibid., 27.

19 Carolyn Raffensperger, "Descansos and Chemicals Policy," Science and Environmental Health Network, June 2008, http://www.sehn.org/web2printer4.php?img=0&lnk=0&page=Volume_13-3.html.

20 Randall Fitzgerald, *The Hundred-Year Lie: How to Protect Yourself from the Chemicals that Are Destroying Your Health* (New York: Plume, 2007), 23.

21 Helena Bottemiller, "FDA Joins Effort to Improve Chemical Screening," Food Safety News, July 22, 2010, http://www.foodsafetynews.com/2010/07/fda-joins-effort-to-improve-chemical-screening.

22 "Swimming in Chemicals," PBS (citing an excerpt from Mark Schapiro, *Exposed: The Toxic Chemistry of Everyday Products and What's at Stake for American Power*), March 21, 2008, http://www.pbs.org/now/shows/412/Exposed-Toxic-Chemistry.html; and Mark Schapiro, *Exposed: The Toxic Chemistry of Everyday Products and What's at Stake for American Power.*

23 "Have you ever counted how many cosmetics or personal care products you use in a day?" Environmental Working Group's Skin Deep Cosmetic Safety Database, http://cosmetic database.com/research/whythismatters.php.

24 Mark Schapiro, *Exposed: The Toxic Chemistry of Everyday Products and What's at Stake for American Power* (White River Junction, VT: Chelsea Green, 2009), 13.

25 Seth Borenstein, "New studies show Americans have scores of toxins in their bodies," Knight Ridder, published on Environmental Working Group website, January 31, 2003, http://www.ewg.org/node/15126.

26 The National Water Quality Inventory: Report to Congress for the 2002 Reporting Cycle. United States Environmental Protection Agency, http://www.epa.gov/305b/2002report/ factsheet2002305b.pdf.

27 Tim Gross, "Plummeting Bee Population Troubling," *Bona Venture*, September 18, 2009, http://media.www.thebv.org/media/storage/paper1111/news/2009/09/18/Opinion/Plum meting.Bee.Population.Troubling-3775364.shtml; and "Saving Bees: What We Know Now," *New York Times*, September 2, 2009, http://roomfordebate.blogs.nytimes.com/ 2009/09/02/saving-bees-what-we-know-now.

Chapter 11: The Mongers

1 Martin Fackler, "At Hiroshima Ceremony, a First for a U.S. Envoy," *New York Times*, August 6, 2010, http://www.nytimes.com/2010/08/07/world/asia/07japan.html; and "Atomic Bombings of Hiroshima and Nagasaki," Wikipedia, http://en.wikipedia.org/wiki/ Atomic_bombings_of_Hiroshima_and_Nagasaki.

2 "Status of World Nuclear Forces 2010," Federation of American Scientists, http://www.fas.org/programs/ssp/nukes/nuclearweapons/nukestatus.html; and "Lists of States with Nuclear Weapons," Wikipedia, http://en.wikipedia.org/wiki/List_of_states_ with_nuclear_weapons.

3 Dwight D. Eisenhower, "Military-Industrial Complex Speech," Public Papers of the Presidents, 1961, http://www.h-net.org/~hst306/documents/indust.html.

4 Elisabeth Bumiller, "The War: A Trillion Can Be Cheap," *New York Times*, July 24, 2010, http://www.nytimes.com/2010/07/25/weekinreview/25bumiller.html.

5 Ibid.

6 "Pentagon's F-35 Fighter Under Fire in Congress," PBS NewsHour transcript, April 21, 2010, http://www.pbs.org/newshour/bb/military/jan-june10/defense_04-21.html?print.

7 Ibid.

8 "What can $611 billion buy?" Boston.com, http://www.boston.com/news/nation/gallery/ 251007war_costs/.

9 "Help End World Hunger," Squidoo, http://www.squidoo.com/world-hunger.

10 "Lockheed Martin spent $3.46 million lobbying in 1Q," Associated Press, June 23, 2010, http://finance.yahoo.com/news/Lockheed-Martin-spent-346-apf-4181942098.html?x=0&.v=2.

11 Alan Simpson, "Political Intelligence," *ComLinks Intel* magazine, October 15, 2004, http:// www.comlinks.com/polintel/pi041015.htm.

12 Dwight D. Eisenhower, "Military-Industrial Complex Speech," Public Papers of the Presidents, 1961, http://www.h-net.org/~hst306/documents/indust.html.

13 Elisabeth Bumiller, "The War: A Trillion Can Be Cheap," *New York Times*, July 24, 2010, http://www.nytimes.com/2010/07/25/weekinreview/25bumiller.html.

14 "2010 Global Peace Index," Institute for Economics and Peace, http://www.visionof humanity.org/wp-content/uploads/2010/06/2010-GPI-Results-and-Methodology-Report1.pdf/PDF/2010/2010%20GPI%20Results%20Report.pdf.

15 "Obama: Nobel Peace Prize is 'call to action,'" CNN Europe, October 9, 2009, http://www.cnn.com/2009/WORLD/europe/10/09/nobel.peace.prize/index.html; and Peter Spiegel, Jonathan Weisman, and Yochi J. Dreazen, "Obama Bets Big on Troop Surge," *Wall Street Journal*, December 2, 2009, http://online.wsj.com/article/NA_WSJ_PUB: SB125967363641871171.html.

16 Russel Goldman and Luis Martinez, "WikiLeaks: At Least 109,000 Killed During Iraq War," ABC News, October 22, 2010, http://abcnews.go.com/Politics/wikileaks-dumps-thousands-classified-military-documents/story?id=11949670.

17 Elisabeth Bumiller, "We Have Met the Enemy and He Is PowerPoint," *New York Times*, April 26, 2010, http://www.nytimes.com/2010/04/27/world/27powerpoint.html?src=tp &pagewanted=print.

18 Ibid.

19 Gordon Lubold and Carol E. Lee, "President Obama: Stanley McChrystal showed 'poor judgment,'" Politico.com, June 22, 2010, http://www.politico.com/news/stories/0610/38837.html

20 Eugene Jarecki, *The American Way of War: Guided Missiles, Misguided Men, and a Republic in Peril* (Free Press, 2008), 94 and 95.

21 Scott Shane and James Dao, "Investigators Study Tangle of Clues on Fort Hood Suspect," *New York Times*, November 14, 2009, http://www.nytimes.com/2009/11/15/us/15hasan.html; and "Gunman Kills 12, Wounds 31 at Fort Hood," NBC News and MSNBC.com, November 5, 2009, http://www.msnbc.msn.com/id/33678801.

22 Scott Shane and James Dao, "Investigators Study Tangle of Clues on Fort Hood Suspect," *New York Times*, November 14, 2009, http://www.nytimes.com/2009/11/15/us/15hasan.htm.

23 "Briton guilty of plotting 'deadly terror attack,'" BBC News, December 10, 2009, http://news.bbc.co.uk/2/hi/uk_news/8404551.stm.

24 Steve Swann, "How British Muslim Adam Khatib Became a Bomb Plotter," BBC News, December 9, 2009, http://news.bbc.co.uk/2/hi/uk_news/8381192.stm.

25 Sabrina Tavernes and Andrew W, Lehren, "A Grim Portrait of Civilian Deaths in Iraq," *The New York Times*, October 22, 2010, http://www.nytimes.com/2010/10/23/world/middleeast/23casualties.html?ref=todayspaper.

26 "U.N.: More than 4 million Iraqis displaced," *Associated Press*, June 5, 2007, http://www.msnbc.msn.com/id/19055852.

27 Robert F. Worth, "Is Yemen the Next Afghanistan?" *New York Times*, July 6, 2010, http://www.nytimes.com/2010/07/11/magazine/11Yemen-t.html.

28 Scott Shane, "Wars Fought and Wars Googled," *New York Times*, June 26, 2010, http://www.nytimes.com/2010/06/27/weekinreview/27shane.html.

29 "Faisal Shahzad," Wikipedia, http://en.wikipedia.org/wiki/Faisal_Shahzad.

30 Dana Priest, "Soldier Suicides at Record Level," *Washington Post*, January 31, 2008, http://www.washingtonpost.com/wp-dyn/content/article/2008/01/30/AR2008013003106.html.

31 Ibid.

32 "1 in 8 returning soldiers suffers from PTSD," Associated Press, June 30, 2004, http://www.msnbc.msn.com/id/5334479.

33 Ronald Glasser, "A Shock Wave of Brain Injuries," *Washington Post*, April 8, 2007, http://www.washingtonpost.com/wpdyn/content/article/2007/04/06/AR2007040601821.html.

34 Dexter Filkins, "Despite Doubt, Karzai Brother Retains Power," *New York Times*, March 30, 2010, http://www.nytimes.com/2010/03/31/world/asia/31karzai.html.

35 Dexter Filkins, "With Troop Pledge, New Demands on Afghans," *New York Times*, December 1, 2009, http://www.nytimes.com/2009/12/02/world/asia/02afghan.html.

36 Anne Gearan, "Mullen says US has Iran strike plan, just in case," Associated Press, August 1, 2010, http://www.washingtontimes.com/news/2010/aug/1/mullen-us-has-iran-strike-plan-just-case/

37 Ibid.

38 Greg Mortenson, *Three Cups of Tea* (New York: Penguin Books, 2007), 268.

39 Nicholas D. Kristof, "One Soldier or 20 Schools," Op-Ed, *New York Times*, July 28, 2010, http://www.nytimes.com/2010/07/29/opinion/29kristof.html.

40 Dwight D. Eisenhower quote, Brainyquote, http://www.brainyquote.com/quotes/quotes/d/dwightdei136898.html.

41 "2010 Global Peace Index," Institute for Economics and Peace," http://www.visionof humanity.org/wp-content/uploads/2010/06/2010-GPI-Results-and-Methodology-Report1.pdf.

42 Charles (Chic) Dambach, *Exhaust the Limits: The Life and Times of a Global Peacebuilder* (Apprentice House, 2010), 274.

Chapter 12: The Sobers

1 Jeanna Bryner, "U.S. Is Richest Nation, But Not Happiest," LiveScience.com, http://www.livescience.com/culture/happiest-nations-income-100701.html.

2 David Michael Bruno, "100 Thing Challenge," GuyNamedDave.com, http://www.guynameddave.com/100-thing-challenge.html.

3 Eckhart Tolle, *A New Earth: Awakening to Your Life's Purpose* (New York: Penguin, 2008), 46.

INTERVIEWS

Albracht, Matthew (Managing Director, The Peace Alliance), interviewed by the authors, August 2010.

Barnard, Neal, M.D. (Clinical Researcher and Author of *Breaking the Food Seduction*), interviewed by authors, May 2010.

Bragman, Howard (Chairman of Fifteen Minutes Public Relations and Author of "Where's my Fifteen Minutes?"), interviewed by the authors, July 2010.

Brown, Leslie, M.D. (Pediatrician and Vegan), interviewed by authors, May 2010.

Cahill, Danny (*Biggest Loser* Star), interviewed by authors, May 2010.

Dambach, Charles F. "Chic" (President and CEO Alliance for Peacebuilding), interviewed by the authors, August 2010.

Guss, Gregory (Licensed Clinical Social Worker), interviewed by the authors, March and June 2010.

Halton, Gene, Ph.D., (Professor of Sociology, University of Notre Dame and Author of "The Great Brain Suck"), interviewed by the authors, May 2010.

Heineke, Becky (Blogger at Overpopulationblog.blogspot.com), interviewed by the authors, June 2010.

Hilton, Perez (Celebrity Blogger, www.perezhilton.com), interviewed by the authors, July 2010.

Jenike, Michael, M.D. (Professor of Psychiatry, Harvard Medical School and Director of the OCD Institute), interviewed by authors, July 2010.

Kasser, Tim (Professor and Chair of Psychology at Knox College and Author of "*The High Price of Materialism*), interviewed by authors, May 2010.

Katherine, Anne (Author of *How to Make Almost Any Diet Work* and *Lick It! Fix Her Appetite Switch*), interviewed by authors, May 2010.

Kucinich, Dennis (Congressman, D-OH), interviewed by the authors, August 2010.

Kuriansky, Judy, Ph.D.(Professional Therapist, Radio Host, and Author of *The Complete Idiots Guide to a Healthy Relationship*), interviewed by the authors, June 2010.

Linn, Susan (Director of Campaign for a Commercial-Free Childhood Commercial-freechildhood.org and Author of "The Case For Make-Believe: Saving Play in a Commercialized World" and "Consuming Kids: Protecting our Children from the Onslaught of Marketing and Advertising"), interviewed by the authors, May 2010.

Mathis, Judge Greg (District Court judge and syndicated television show judge), interviewed by the authors, March 2010.

Pratt, Travis (Author of *Addicted to Incarceration—Corrections Policy and the Politics of Misinformation in the United States* and Associate Professor, School of Criminology and Criminal Justice Arizona State University), interviewed by the authors, March 2010.

Roskos, Laura, Ph.D., (Co-President of U. S. Section Women's International League for Peace and Freedom), interviewed by the authors, August 2010.

Samuels, Howard, Psy D. (Licensed Clinical Psychologist, Psychotherapist, Founder and CEO of The Hills Treatment Center in LA), interviewed by the authors, March 2010.

Samuels, Howard, Psy D. (Licensed Clinical Psychologist, Psychotherapist, and Founder and CEO of The Hills Treatment Center in Los Angeles), interviewed by the authors, March 2010.

Seeley, Ken (Addiction Expert and Founder of Intervention 911), interviewed by the authors, March 2010.

Selman, Donna (Author of *Punishment for Sale* and Associate Professor of Criminology, at Eastern Michigan University), interviewed by the authors, March 2010.

Soffer, Simeon (Director of *Fight to The Max*), interviewed by the authors, March 2010.

Switalski, Erin (Executive Director, Women's Voices for the Earth), interviewed by authors, July 2010.

Triessl, Alison (Attorney and Co-Founder/CEO of Pasadena Recovery Center), interviewed by the authors, April 2010.

Andrea (Anonymous Cleaning Addict/Clean Freak), interviewed by authors, July 2010.

April East (Anonymous Gaming Addict), interviewed by authors, July 2010.

Interviews recorded by phone with permission.

INDEX

ABOUT THE AUTHORS

Jane Velez-Mitchell is an award-winning television journalist and host of the hit TV show *Issues with Jane Velez-Mitchell* on HLN. She is the author of the *New York Times* bestselling memoir *iWant*, which outlines her journey from alcoholism and overconsumption to a simpler, honest life. With more than a decade and a half of sobriety, Velez-Mitchell has become a nationally recognized voice on addiction, often commenting on the subject for CNN, Tru TV, and other cable networks. With more than three decades of journalistic experience, Velez-Mitchell is an astute observer of national trends.

Sandra Mohr is an award-winning filmmaker who wrote, directed, and produced *Stock Shock,* a powerful documentary about stock market manipulation. Coauthor of *Addict Nation,* Mohr also assisted Velez-Mitchell with her books *Secrets Can Be Murder* and *iWant.* Her company, Mohr Productions, Inc., creates programming/commercials for TV and the Internet.